Clinicians' Guides to Radionuclide Hybrid Imaging

PET/CT

Series Editors

Jamshed B. Bomanji
London, UK

Gopinath Gnanasegaran
London, UK

Stefano Fanti
Bologna, Italy

Homer A. Macapinlac
Houston, Texas, USA

Hybrid imaging with PET/CT and SPECT/CT provides high-quality information on function and structure, thereby permitting accurate localization, characterization, and diagnosis. There is extensive evidence to support the value of PET/CT, which has made a significant impact on oncological imaging and the management of patients with cancer. The evidence in favor of SPECT/CT, especially for orthopaedic indications, is evolving and increasing. This pocket book series on hybrid imaging (PET/CT and SPECT/CT) is specifically aimed at referring clinicians, nuclear medicine/radiology physicians, radiographers/technologists, and nurses who routinely work in nuclear medicine and participate in multidisciplinary meetings. The series will include 18 pocket books on PET/CT and 3 on SPECT/CT. Compiled under the auspices of the British Nuclear Medicine Society, the series is the joint work of many colleagues and professionals worldwide who share a common vision and purpose in promoting and supporting nuclear medicine as an important imaging specialty for the diagnosis and management of oncological and non-oncological conditions.

The PET/CT pocket book series will be dedicated to some of the Society's recently departed peers, including Prof Ignac Fogelman, Dr Muriel Buxton-Thomas and Prof Ajit K Padhy

More information about this series at http://www.springer.com/series/13803

Dragana Sobic Saranovic • Mariza Vorster
Sanjay Gambhir • Thomas Neil Pascual
Editors

PET/CT in Tuberculosis

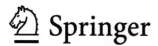

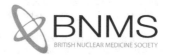

Editors
Dragana Sobic Saranovic
Center for Nuclear Medicine,
Clinical Center of Serbia
Faculty of Medicine University of Belgrade
Belgrade
Serbia

Sanjay Gambhir
Deptartment of Nuclear Medicine
Sanjay Gandhi Post Graduate Institute
of Lucknow
Lucknow
India

Mariza Vorster
Department of Nuclear Medicine
University of Pretoria
Pretoria
South Africa

Thomas Neil Pascual
Nuclear Medicine and Diagnostic Imaging
International Atomic Energy Agency
Wien-Vereinte Nationen
Wien
Austria

ISSN 2367-2439   ISSN 2367-2447 (electronic)
Clinicians' Guides to Radionuclide Hybrid Imaging - PET/CT
ISBN 978-3-030-47008-1   ISBN 978-3-030-47009-8   (eBook)
https://doi.org/10.1007/978-3-030-47009-8

This Springer imprint is published by the registered company Springer Nature Switzerland AG
The registered company address is: Gewerbestrasse 11, 6330 Cham, Switzerland

PET/CT series is dedicated to Prof Ignac Fogelman, Dr Muriel Buxton-Thomas and Prof Ajit K. Padhy

Foreword

Clear and concise clinical indications for PET/CT in the management of the oncology and non-oncology patient are presented in this series of 15 separate booklets.

The impact on better staging, tailored management and specific treatment of the patient with cancer has been achieved with the advent of this multimodality imaging technology. Early and accurate diagnosis will always pay, and clear information can be gathered with PET/CT on treatment responses. Prognostic information is gathered and can forward guide additional therapeutic options.

It is a fortunate coincidence that PET/CT was able to derive great benefit from radionuclide-labelled probes, which deliver good and often excellent target to non-target signals. Whilst labelled glucose remains the cornerstone for the clinical benefit achieved, a number of recent probes are definitely adding benefit. PET/CT is hence an evolving technology, extending its applications and indications. Significant advances in the instrumentation and data processing available have also contributed to this technology, which delivers high throughput and a wealth of data, with good patient tolerance and indeed patient and public acceptance. As an example, the role of PET/CT in the evaluation of cardiac disease is also covered, with emphasis on labelled rubidium and labelled glucose studies.

The novel probes of labelled choline; labelled peptides, such as DOTATATE; and, most recently, labelled prostate-specific membrane antigen (PSMA) have gained rapid clinical utility and acceptance, as significant PET/CT tools for the management of neuroendocrine disease and prostate cancer patients, notwithstanding all the advances achieved with other imaging modalities, such as MRI. Hence, a chapter reviewing novel PET tracers forms a part of this series.

The oncological community has recognised the value of PET/CT and has delivered advanced diagnostic criteria for some of the most important indications for PET/CT. This includes the recent Deauville criteria for the classification of PET/CT patients with lymphoma—similar criteria are expected to develop for other malignancies, such as head and neck cancer, melanoma and pelvic malignancies. For completion, a separate section covers the role of PET/CT in radiotherapy planning, discussing the indications for planning biological tumour volumes in relevant cancers.

These booklets offer simple, rapid and concise guidelines on the utility of PET/CT in a range of oncological indications. They also deliver a rapid aide-memoire on the merits and appropriate indications for PET/CT in oncology.

London, UK   Peter J. Ell, FMedSci, DR HC, AΩA

Preface

Tuberculosis remains the leading infectious disease cause of death worldwide despite advances in diagnosis and treatment. It primarily affects the lungs; however, extrapulmonary tuberculosis can also occur in approximately 15% of new cases. In these settings, diagnostic imaging, especially PET/CT, can play an important role in better evaluation of the disease.

This aim of this book is to present the updates in epidemiology, clinical presentation, diagnosis, and management of tuberculosis. The main part of the book is dedicated to the state of the art in diagnostic imaging, with special attention drawn to PET/CT imaging in tuberculosis. The book covers principles of PET/CT, FDG, and non-FDG radiopharmaceuticals used for evaluation of tuberculosis, practical aspects of patient preparation and imaging protocols, PET/CT findings in diagnosis and follow-up of pulmonary and extrapulmonary tuberculosis, and evaluation of treatment response. PET/CT findings in the presence of frequent coinfection with HIV/AIDS, possible pitfalls, mimics of tuberculosis, and limitations of PET/CT are also presented.

This book is a multidisciplinary approach and joint effort of physicians from six countries gathered together in IAEA Coordinated Research Project on the role of PET/CT in extrapulmonary tuberculosis, E15021.

The book is intended for referring clinicians, nuclear medicine and radiology physicians, medical students, radiographers, technologists, and nurses who work in nuclear medicine department.

Belgrade, Serbia   Dragana Sobic Saranovic
Pretoria, South Africa   Mariza Vorster
Lucknow, India   Sanjay Gambhir
Wien, Austria   Thomas Neil Pascual

Acknowledgements

The series co-ordinators and editors would like to express sincere gratitude to the members of the British Nuclear Medicine Society, patients, teachers, colleagues, students, the industry and the BNMS Education Committee Members, for their continued support and inspiration.

Andy Bradley
Brent Drake
Francis Sundram
James Ballinger
Parthiban Arumugam
Rizwan Syed
Sai Han
Vineet Prakash

Contents

Tuberculosis: A General Overview

1

K. M. G. Mokoala and A. O. Ankrah

Contents

K. M. G. Mokoala
Department of Nuclear Medicine, Steve Biko Academic Hospital, University of Pretoria, Pretoria, South Africa

A. O. Ankrah (✉)
Department of Nuclear Medicine, Steve Biko Academic Hospital, University of Pretoria, Pretoria, South Africa

Department of Nuclear Medicine and Molecular Imaging, University Medical Center Groningen, University of Groningen, Groningen, Netherlands

National Centre for Radiotherapy and Nuclear Medicine, Korle Bu Teaching Hospital, Accra, Ghana

© Springer Nature Switzerland AG 2020
D. Sobic Saranovic et al. (eds.), *PET/CT in Tuberculosis*, Clinicians' Guides to Radionuclide Hybrid Imaging, https://doi.org/10.1007/978-3-030-47009-8_1

1

1.1   Introduction

Tuberculosis (TB) is a disease that humans have been grappling with for centuries, with paleohistological studies demonstrating that TB has afflicted humankind from as early as 8000 BC or even earlier [1]. In 1882, the German scientist Robert Heinrich Koch first identified the causative organism for TB, *Mycobacterium tuberculosis* (*M. tuberculosis*). *M. tuberculosis* is part of the *M. tuberculosis* complex that consists of *Mycobacterium* species causing disease in humans or animals. Other species in the M. tuberculosis complex include *M. africanum, M. bovis, M. microti* and *M. canetti* [2].

1.1.1   Epidemiology

Despite the fact that TB is both curable and preventable, it remains one of the top ten causes of mortality worldwide and has overtaken human immunodeficiency virus (HIV) as the leading cause of mortality from a single infectious agent [3]. In 2017, TB was responsible for the death of nearly 1.3 million HIV-negative people and of approximately 300,000 HIV-positive people. Globally, roughly 10 million people (mostly adults) developed TB in 2017. In patients 15 years or older, males were affected twice as often as females and 10% were under 15 years [3]. Nine percent of all patients who developed TB in 2017 also had HIV infection.

1.1.2   Geographic Distribution

TB affects every region in the world. In 2017, most of the new TB cases occurred in Southeast Asia and Western Pacific regions (62%) followed by the African region (25%). There has been a trend change in newly reported cases with most developed countries now demonstrating a significant decline in the disease burden from TB, while in developing or low-income countries TB remains a significant health problem. The majority (72%) of new cases of TB coinfected with HIV in 2017 occurred in Africa.

1.2   Risk Factors for Active TB (Progression from Latent TB Infection)

Approximately 23% of the world is infected with TB without clinical or radiologic evidence of disease in a state known as "latent TB infection" (LTBI). Of all patients infected with *M. tuberculosis*, only a small proportion (5–10%) will develop active disease. People living with HIV, those with a weakened immune system caused by prolonged use of medicines (steroid or TNF-α inhibitors), diabetes mellitus, renal insufficiency, and silicosis (to name a few) are at a higher risk of falling ill from TB. Socioeconomic status remains a significant risk factor because TB is a disease of poverty that thrives where overcrowding and malnutrition are prevalent. Other risk factors include heavy alcohol consumption and smoking.

1.3 Clinical Presentation

Although the lung is the primary site affected by TB, it can cause disease in any organ, and is included in the differential diagnosis of a vast range of clinical presentations. The nonspecific constitutional symptoms of fever, weight loss, and night sweat together with the disease site-specific complaints are used to guide further workup and management. The features commonly associated with active pulmonary TB are a cough, hemoptysis, chest pain, and fatigue. Symptoms of TB meningitis may include the following: headache (persistent for 2–3 weeks or intermittent) and subtle changes in the mental status that may progress to coma. In skeletal TB, patients may present with back pain or stiffness, lower extremity paralysis, or arthritis (usually involving one joint, most often the hip or knee, followed by the ankle, elbow, wrist, and shoulder). In elderly patients, those with HIV coinfection and extrapulmonary TB may present with nonspecific symptoms and signs. Health workers should have a high index of suspicion for TB when dealing with HIV-positive patients since the risk of disease is high, and the diagnosis is difficult. Patients with low CD4 counts indicating suppressed immunity are at an increased risk for both extrapulmonary and disseminated disease [2].

1.4 Physical Examination

The clinical manifestation of the disease will depend on the organs involved. Patients with pulmonary TB may have abnormal breath sounds, especially in the lung apices. If there is lung consolidation, there may be rales or bronchial breathing. If a pleural effusion is present, the breaths sounds may be diminished or absent. TB lymphadenopathy is among the most frequent presentations of extrapulmonary TB. Tuberculosis is responsible for 43–64% of peripheral lymphadenopathy in the developing world [4, 5]. It presents as swelling of one or more lymph nodes and is usually bilateral, typically involving the cervical chain (anterior and posterior) or supraclavicular lymph nodes. Other signs of extrapulmonary TB would depend on the site involved. Importantly, the absence of physical findings on examination does not exclude active TB.

1.5 Diagnosis

Early and accurate diagnosis of TB, HIV-associated TB, and drug-resistant TB is vital in order to initiate appropriate therapy promptly. Early and appropriate treatment prevents morbidity and mortality from this curable disease and also minimizes its spread. The diagnosis of TB can often be complicated and is made more difficult by the lack of accurate and rapid diagnostics. A formal diagnosis requires bacteriological confirmation; however, in some cases clinical features are used to make the diagnosis. Bacteriological confirmation was available in only 56% of the 5.5 million new and relapsing pulmonary TB patients notified globally in 2017. In the remaining patients, the diagnosis of TB was made based on symptoms, chest radiography abnormalities, suggestive histology, or a combination of the aforementioned [3].

The best biological sample to stain and culture *M. tuberculosis* for pulmonary TB is freshly prepared expectorate. There are, however, circumstances where it is impossible to get sputum, and bronchial aspirates or bronchoalveolar lavage fluid may be used for the analysis. Acid-fast staining is a rapid and inexpensive screening test for acid-fast bacilli and remains the main method used for diagnosis of TB in many countries. Culture-based methods of diagnosis are the current reference standard, but they require developed laboratories where results may take up to 12 weeks. Whenever the culture is positive for TB, drug susceptibility of the *M. tuberculosis* isolated should be done. Awaiting results should not delay the start of therapy and empiric treatment, and first-line anti-TB drugs should be initiated while waiting for the culture results. The use of Xpert® MTB/RIF assay, a rapid molecular testing which can diagnose TB within 2 h and also determine drug resistance, is gradually becoming the preferred method of diagnosing TB. Xpert® MTB/RIF has a much better accuracy than a sputum smear, and results are available much faster than culture results which may take up to 12 weeks to become available.

1.5.1 Other Investigations

In pulmonary TB, a chest radiograph should be obtained to evaluate for possible associated pulmonary findings such as cavitations, calcified infiltrates, or nodules. Other imaging procedures, such as computed tomography (CT) scans, may provide better definition of some of the lesions noted on chest radiograph such as cavitations and infiltrates. In extrapulmonary TB, the suspected affected site will guide the investigation. The test may be as simple and noninvasive such as a urinalysis to screen for genitourinary TB (sterile pyuria) to more invasive procedures such as a lumbar puncture to obtain CSF or a deep tissue biopsy.

1.5.2 Diagnosis of Latent Tuberculosis Infection (LTBI)

Screening for LTBI involves the use of the Mantoux tuberculin skin test with purified protein derivative (PPD). Blood tests based on interferon-gamma release assay (IGRA) with antigens specific for *M. tuberculosis* can also detect latent infection [6]. These tests may be false-positive in a patient with previous bacillus Calmette-Guérin (BCG) vaccination (more frequently with the Mantoux test) or false-negative in a patient with severe immunosuppression [7].

1.5.3 Challenges in TB Diagnosis

Childhood, sputum smear-negative pulmonary, and extrapulmonary TB remain some of the most significant diagnostic challenges [2]. The most common causes of delay in diagnosis are HIV coinfection, socioeconomic factors, stigma, time to reach healthcare facilities, and visiting more than one healthcare provider before diagnosis [7]. A non-sputum blood-based 3-gene signature score appears to be a promising tool for assessing the progression of latent to active TB, for detection of active disease, monitoring of anti-TB treatment, and evaluation of residual TB after completion of treatment [7].

1.6   Special Categories

1.6.1 TB and HIV

The HIV pandemic has amplified the global burden of TB, particularly in Sub-Saharan Africa [8]. In the coinfected host, the infections have a synergistic deleterious effect on the host, accelerating the deterioration of immunological functions and resulting in premature death if untreated. HIV coinfection is the most potent known risk factor for the progression of *M. tuberculosis* infection, increasing the risk of latent TB reactivation 20- to 40-fold. Tuberculosis, on the other hand, has been reported to exacerbate HIV infection, causing it to progress [8]. Patients at any stage of HIV may get TB, and the manifestation of TB depends primarily on the level of immunosuppression. Early during HIV disease, symptoms and signs are similar to those in HIV-uninfected individuals. As the HIV progresses symptoms become atypical [9].

1.6.1.1 Immune Reconstitution TB
Immune reconstitution as a result of combined antiretroviral therapy may "unmask" previously asymptomatic TB, and this is known as tuberculosis-associated immune reconstitution inflammatory syndrome (TB-IRIS). TB-IRIS may also present as a "paradoxical" worsening of the disease (TB) during anti-TB therapy. Approximately one-third of HIV-associated TB cases present with TB-IRIS. Extrapulmonary disease (disseminated TB or TB lymphadenitis), low CD4 cell counts, and earlier initiation of antiretroviral therapy (ART) after tuberculosis treatment are factors associated with an increased risk for TB-IRIS [10].

1.6.1.2 Drug-Resistant TB
Drug resistance poses a severe challenge to public health and clinical management of TB. The risk factors for developing resistance are intermittent drug use, errors in medical prescription, poor patient adherence, and low-quality TB drugs [3, 11, 12]. The most potent risk factor for resistance to second-line drugs is a previous and

mainly incorrect use of these drugs. There has been an increase in drug sensitivity testing worldwide. In 2017, 2 million (30%) of the 6.7 million new and previously treated TB patients notified globally were tested for Rifampicin resistance [3]. In addition, 82% of TB cases found to be resistant to rifampicin were also resistant to isoniazid. Resistance to both rifampicin and isoniazid is referred to as multidrug resistant TB (MDR-TB). Globally 160,684 cases of MDR-TB were detected and notified in 2017. A total of 10,800 cases of from TB from 77 countries were found to be extensively drug resistant, with 88% of cases being in WHO European and Southeast Asia regions [3]. Extensively drug-resistant TB is unresponsive to second-line anti-TB drug fluoroquinolone and an injectable drug over and above multidrug-resistant TB.

1.6.1.3 TB in Children

TB remains a significant but often unrecognized cause of disease and death among children in areas where the disease is endemic [13, 14]. Poor case ascertainment and incomplete recording and reporting limit the accuracy of disease burden estimates in children [15–17]. HIV coinfection has had a significant impact on the epidemiology of TB in children, especially in sub-Saharan Africa. Young women of childbearing age are more likely to be affected by both entities. This has resulted in high rates of exposure to tuberculosis among infants born to mothers who are HIV positive and in the high rates of tuberculosis among infants infected with HIV [18].

Children are usually investigated for TB after presenting with symptoms or signs suggestive of the disease, as a result of contact investigation, or during routine immigration screening. TB diagnosis in children is complicated due to the diversity of the clinical presentation and the nonspecific nature of the symptoms. Chest radiography is one of the most useful diagnostic tools to guide the diagnosis [13].

Bacteriological confirmation remains the ultimate goal. However, confirmation rates are low. In the immunologically vulnerable children, treatment must be initiated promptly and not delayed if the clinical suspicion for TB is high [13, 16].

1.7 Future Developments

Novel diagnostic tools such as whole-body imaging with positron emission tomography (PET)/computerized tomography (CT) may help to address some of the challenges encountered in the management of TB by detecting sites of extrapulmonary involvement, directing biopsies, monitoring of treatment response, determining the extent of disease involvement, and possibly predicting which individuals are more likely to develop drug-resistant TB or to progress from latent to active TB.

1.8 Conclusion

Tuberculosis continues to affect every part of the world, despite being both curable and preventable, with low-income countries disproportionately affected. It can infect people at any age and affect any organ system, while its diagnosis in children, extrapulmonary TB, and HIV-associated TB can be challenging. Drug-resistant TB further adds to the challenges in managing this infection. New diagnostic tools are urgently needed for the comprehensive management of this deadly infection.

References

1. Baker O, Lee OY, Wu HH, Besra GS, Minnikin DE, Llewellyn G, et al. Human tuberculosis predates domestication in ancient Syria. Tuberculosis (Edinb). 2015;95(Suppl 1):S4–S12.
2. Lawn SD, Zumla AI. Tuberculosis. Lancet. 2011;378(9785):57–72.
3. World Health Organization. Global tuberculosis report 2018. Geneva: World Health Organization; 2018. In: World Health Organization, editor. France 2018.
4. Dandapat MC, Mishra BM, Dash SP, Kar PK. Peripheral lymph node tuberculosis: a review of 80 cases. Br J Surg. 1990;77(8):911–2.
5. Jha BC, Dass A, Nagarkar NM, Gupta R, Singhal S. Cervical tuberculous lymphadenopathy: changing clinical pattern and concepts in management. Postgrad Med J. 2001;77(905):185–7.
6. Caufield NL. Diagnosis of active tuberculosis disease: from microscopy to molecular techniques. J Clin Tuberc Other Mycobact Dis. 2016;4:33–43.
7. Storla DG, Yimer S, Bjune GA. A systematic review of delay in the diagnosis and treatment of tuberculosis. BMC Public Health. 2008;8:15.
8. Pawlowski A, Jansson M, Skold M, Rottenberg ME, Kallenius G. Tuberculosis and HIV co-infection. PLoS Pathog. 2012;8(2):e1002464.
9. Gray JM, Cohn DL. Tuberculosis and HIV coinfection. Semin Respir Crit Care Med. 2013;34(1):32–43.
10. Colebunders R, John L, Huyst V, Kambugu A, Scano F, Lynen L. Tuberculosis immune reconstitution inflammatory syndrome in countries with limited resources. Int J Tuberc Lung Dis. 2006;10(9):946–53.
11. Glaziou P, Floyd K, Raviglione MC. Global epidemiology of tuberculosis. Semin Respir Crit Care Med. 2018;39(3):271–85.
12. Matteelli A, Roggi A, Carvalho AC. Extensively drug-resistant tuberculosis: epidemiology and management. Clin Epidemiol. 2014;6:111–8.
13. Perez-Velez CM, Marais BJ. Tuberculosis in children. N Engl J Med. 2012;367(4):348–61.
14. Perez-Velez CM, Roya-Pabon CL, Marais BJ. A systematic approach to diagnosing intrathoracic tuberculosis in children. J Infect. 2017;74(Suppl 1):S74–83.
15. Newton SM, Brent AJ, Anderson S, Whittaker E, Kampmann B. Paediatric tuberculosis. Lancet Infect Dis. 2008;8(8):498–510.
16. Britton P, Perez-Velez CM, Marais BJ. Diagnosis, treatment and prevention of tuberculosis in children. N S W Public Health Bull. 2013;24(1):15–21.
17. Marais BJ. Tuberculosis in children. J Paediatr Child Health. 2014;50(10):759–67.
18. Bruchfeld J, Correia-Neves M, Kallenius G. Tuberculosis and HIV coinfection. Cold Spring Harb Perspect Med. 2015;5(7):a017871.

Diagnosis of Tuberculosis: Microbiological and Imaging Perspective

2

Sanjay Gambhir, Kasturi Rangan, and Manish Ora

Contents

2.1   Introduction

Tuberculosis has been in global limelight since 1990s [1] and was declared as global emergency in 1993. India has been the frontrunner in the incidence of tuberculosis, carting a burden of 27% of all the TB cases in the world. TB is one of the top 10 causes of death worldwide [2]. In 2017, TB caused an estimated 1.3 million deaths and 10 million people (range, 9.0–11.1 million) developed TB disease globally [2]. In 2014, world health assembly pledged a strategy to end tuberculosis with a goal of achieving reduction of incidence of TB globally by less than 50%, and reducing mortality by less than 75% by 2025, 90% in 2030, and 95% in 2035, respectively [2]. Ending TB globally could yield US$ 1.2 trillion overall economic return on investments [2].

S. Gambhir (✉) · K. Rangan · M. Ora
Department of Nuclear Medicine, S.G.P.G.I.M.S, Lucknow, India

© Springer Nature Switzerland AG 2020
D. Sobic Saranovic et al. (eds.), *PET/CT in Tuberculosis*, Clinicians' Guides to Radionuclide Hybrid Imaging, https://doi.org/10.1007/978-3-030-47009-8_2

The goal of definitive treatment can only be possible if the diagnosis is precise and on time. Tuberculosis is always a diagnostic challenge due to dynamism in its pathogenesis and wide-ranging presentations. Diagnosis of TB is certain when there is a definite evidence of bacteria. TB tests used for diagnosis look directly for the bacteria or their contents, whereas radiological tests look at the secondary effects of tubercular infection.

The emergence of TB drug resistance, TB in children, and TB in immunocompromised patients have added to the challenges in the diagnosis, and there is a need for urgent implementation of better technology to combat vengeance of the disease.

2.1.1   Investigations—Microbiological Tests

Various tests are available to diagnose TB as well as to know the susceptibility of the TB bacteria to antitubercular drugs (ATT). TB diseases which are not susceptible to first-line ATT are called drug-resistant TB. Some of the TB tests are skin test, culture test, TB interferon-gamma release assays (IGRAs), sputum smear microscopy, fluorescent microscopy, molecular tests (GeneXpert and TrueNat), and drug susceptibility tests. We briefly explain each test for basic understanding.

2.1.1.1 Mantoux Tuberculin Skin Test
It is used to check for latent TB infection, but in countries with high incidence of TB infection it often leads to high false-positive results. A small amount of the tuberculin is injected into the skin and examined after 48–72 h. The test results depend on the size of the induration or swelling.

2.1.1.2 Interferon-Gamma Release Assays (IGRAs)
IGRAs are blood tests that measure a person's immune response to the mycobacteria, and thus help in the detection of latent tuberculosis. If the patient is infected with *M. tuberculosis*, their white blood cells will release interferon (IFN)-gamma in response to contact with the TB antigens. Detection of interferons (a type of cytokine) released by immune system forms the basis of IGRA tests. IGRAs are FDA approved and available as QuantiFERON TB gold and T-SPOT TB tests [3]. Blood samples are taken from the patient and results can be obtained within 24 h.

2.1.1.3 Sputum Smear Microscopy
It is the first test done in countries with high rate of incidence. Sputum is smeared as a thin layer on a glass slide and examined for TB bacteria using special stains such as Ziehl–Neelsen stain. Bacteria are seen as elongated purple rods in blue background. It is fairly quick and cheap. However, the sensitivity is only 50–60% [4].

2.1.1.4 Fluorescent Microscopy
The smear can be seen through a halogen or mercury vapor lamp, allowing broader and rapid examination of the smear. World Health Organization (WHO) had recommended to switch to LED microscopy instead of conventional light microscope.

Fluorescent microscopy (FM) is about 10% more sensitive than light microscopy [5]. Recent development of a tablet camera attached to an optical chamber with LED filters has been used to read slides. The device has shown sensitivities within 15% of LED-FM devices [6].

2.1.1.5 Mycobacterial Culture

Cultures are gold standard for TB diagnosis and drug sensitivity testing (DST). The Löwenstein–Jensen medium, more commonly known as LJ medium, is a growth medium for culture of *Mycobacterium tuberculosis*. Major drawback is that the test takes 6–8 weeks to yield a result, needs trained personnel for monitoring and reporting, and requires a biosafety level 3 environment.

Liquid cultures are turning out to be more sensitive and yield rapid results within 2 weeks [7]. Automated liquid culture platforms, specifically the mycobacterial growth indicator tube BD BACTEC MGIT (BD Diagnostics, New Jersey, USA), which has been examined by the WHO for drug-susceptibility testing (DST), scans processed specific sputum bottles and determines MTB growth by measuring oxygen depletion [8].

2.1.1.6 Molecular Test

- *Nucleic acid amplification test (NAA)*—Nucleic acid amplification tests (NAATs) amplify genome-specific targets, through different methods: polymerase chain reaction (PCR), transcription-mediated amplification (TMA), loop-mediated amplification (LAMP), nucleic acid sequence-based amplification (NASBA), and strand displacement amplification (SDA).
- *Line probe assay*—Line probe assays were the first TB NAATs to be endorsed by the WHO in 2008. They extract genomic DNA, then select DNA targets, and label them with biotin to create amplicons. The amplicons are then applied to a strip with specific oligonucleotide probes. Subsequently, bounded amplicons are detected through attachment of a label and the visualization of a dark band against a scoring chart. These assays allow for identification of mutations, which aids in drug-susceptibility testing. They are useful to detect drug susceptibility rapidly. Resistance to INH occur primarily due to *katG* mutation, followed by mutation at InhA active site [9]. Mutation in pro B region are found in about 96% of rifampicin-resistant *M. tuberculosis*. Sensitivity and specificity crosses >90% for both resistance detection [9]. Currently, the Genotype MTBDRplus assay is endorsed by the WHO for rapid detection of MDR-TB in smear-positive samples and culture isolates.
- *Microarray platform*—It is able to distinguish between MTB and *Mycobacterium avium* through the use of a single-tube PCR reaction, which incorporates a fluorescent label to facilitate visualization.
- *Xpert MTB/RIF*—It is rapid, automated, and cartilage-based NAA that can detect TB along with rifampicin resistance. The GeneXpert cartridges are preloaded with all of the necessary reagents for sample processing, DNA extraction, amplification, and laser detection of the amplified *rpo B* gene target. A major advantage of the Xpert MTB/RIF test is that it can be accurately administrated with

minimal hands-on technical time. While it should be noted that mono-resistance to rifampicin is found in approximately 5% of rifampicin-resistant strains, a high proportion of rifampicin resistance is associated with concurrent resistance to isoniazid (~95%) [10]. Thus, detecting resistance to rifampicin can be used as a marker for MDR-TB with a high level of accuracy.

2.1.1.7 Drug Sensitivity Testing

Microscopically observed drug susceptibility (MODS), a manual culture assay, has been shown to perform as well as automated liquid culture systems, and can be used as a rapid test to identify MTB and resistance to RIF and INH [11]. Other manual noncommercial tests include colorimetric redox indicator (CRI), nitrate reductase assay (NRA), and the thin-layer agar (TLA) assay. The limitations of these noncommercial tests are that users require extensive training in order to ensure standardization and quality, rendering scalability impractical.

2.1.1.8 Biomarker Tests

Non-sputum TB tests are available for diagnosing pediatric, extrapulmonary, and immunocompromised patients. Obtaining sputum from these patients is difficult [12]. Also existing serological, antibody tests have been shown to lack accuracy and are discouraged by the WHO [13]. Further research is important in this area, as serological tests might open the door for a simple, rapid, and lateral flow test.

Antigen detection might hold some promise (e.g., lipoarabinomannan (LAM) in urine). The Alere Determine TB LAM Ag rapid test allows for detection of LAM and aids in the detection of TB in HIV. However, LAM assays have low sensitivity in patients with CD4 counts greater than 200 cells/μl [14], and their use is not endorsed by the WHO.

Volatile organic compounds (VOCs) allow for the detection of early MTB infections through breath. The use of VOCs might allow for improved diagnosis of MTB in children and in HIV patients. Biomarkers including adenosine deaminase (ADA) and free interferon gamma (IFN-g) have the potential to detect TB, especially pleural TB.

2.1.1.9 Challenges for Microbiological Diagnosis

1. Highly TB-burdened countries do not have access to effective diagnosis. In spite of availability of high-end diagnostic tools, many of them are not accessible due to financial constraints.
2. Limitations are also associated with existing diagnostic capacity in detecting extrapulmonary tuberculosis (EPTB), pediatric TB, people living with HIV, and newer drug resistance.

2.1.2   Imaging in TB

Imaging plays a major role in diagnosis of tuberculosis. It not only detects the abnormality caused by the pathological process, but also guides the clinician to perform biopsy, help in follow-up, and determine the therapeutic end point.

TB is considered to be a chameleon in imaging perspective, as it has varied appearances in various organs. Although the thorax is most frequently involved site, it may involve any organ systems (e.g., the respiratory, central nervous, musculoskeletal, gastrointestinal, genitourinary systems, others).

2.1.2.1 Pulmonary Tuberculosis

Pulmonary tuberculosis has been divided into primary and postprimary tuberculosis on the basis of time of exposure.

Primary Tuberculosis: It is seen in patients not previously exposed to *M. tuberculosis*. Primary tuberculosis manifests as four main entities: parenchymal disease, lymphadenopathy, miliary disease, and pleural effusion.

Chest X-ray—It has high sensitivity for TB (~80%), but modest specificity (~70%), as many lung diseases can cause similar X-ray abnormalities [15]. Therefore, chest X-ray is a very good triage or screening tool and can identify those who require confirmatory testing. Radiographic tools are being revolutionized in two certain ways: first, through the use of digital plates and digital radiography, and second through computer-aided diagnosis [16]. Direct digital radiography consists of a digital detector which replaces the plates present in conventional radiography; computer radiography involves a specific plate which produces an analog signal allowing the image to be digitized and stored on a dedicated computer [17].

1. *Parenchymal Disease*—Typically, parenchymal disease manifests as dense, homogeneous parenchymal consolidation in any lobe. In adults it predominantly involves lower and middle lobes. In two-thirds of cases, the parenchymal focus resolves without sequelae at conventional radiograph (Fig. 2.1).
2. *Lymphadenopathy (LNDs)*—Radiographic evidence of lymphadenopathy is seen in most of the children and half of adults. Any nodes greater than 2 cm with central necrosis at CT are highly suggestive of active disease [18]. CT is more sensitive than chest radiography for LNDs.

Fig. 2.1 Axial CT section—Consolidatory changes are noted in posterior segment of the right upper lobe

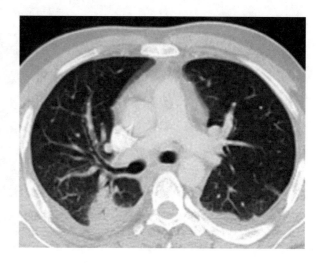

3. *Miliary Disease*—Clinically significant miliary disease affects between 1% and 7% of patients with all forms of tuberculosis [19]. It is usually seen in the elderly, infants, and immunocompromised persons, manifesting within 6 months of initial exposure. High-resolution CT is more sensitive than conventional radiography (Fig. 2.2).

4. *Pleural Effusion*—A pleural effusion is seen in approximately one-fourth of patients with proved primary tuberculosis [19]. The effusion may be the sole manifestation of tuberculosis and usually manifests 3–7 months after initial exposure. It is uncommon in infants. It is usually unilateral, and may cause complications (e.g., empyema formation, fistulization, bone erosion, etc.). Ultrasonography (US) often demonstrates a complex septate effusion and helps in guiding diagnostic/therapeutic tapping (Fig. 2.3).

2.1.2.2 Postprimary Tuberculosis

Postprimary tuberculosis remains primarily a disease of young adult and adulthood. It occurs in patients previously sensitized to *M tuberculosis*. Primary tuberculosis is usually self-limiting, whereas postprimary tuberculosis is progressive, with cavitation as its main feature. It may result in hematogenous dissemination of the disease as well as disease spread throughout the lungs. Healing usually occurs with fibrosis and calcification.

• Parenchymal Disease (Fig. 2.4)—The initial finding in parenchymal disease is patchy, poorly defined consolidation, particularly in the apical and posterior segments of the upper lobes [15]. In the majority of cases, more than one pulmonary segment is generally involved with no distinct separation.

• Cavitation, the hallmark feature of postprimary tuberculosis, affects nearly 50% of patients. The cavities typically have thick, irregular marginated walls, which become smooth and thin with successful treatment. Upon resolution they can result in emphysematous change or scarring (Figs. 2.7 and 2.8). In case of endobronchial spread of infection, tree-in-bud opacities can be seen. It is usually seen

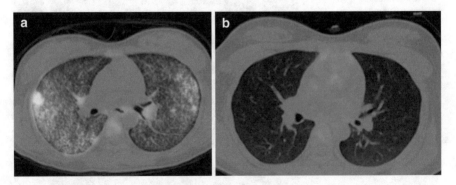

Fig. 2.2 Axial sections of 18 F-FDG PET–CT(pre- and post-therapy), (**a**) image reveals extensive FDG-avid miliary lung nodules with a patch of consolidation and multiple tree in bud opacities. (**b**) Image reveals normal lung parenchyma after anti-tubercular treatment for 6 months

Fig. 2.3 Axial CT section—Right pleural effusion with bilateral hilar lymphadenopathy

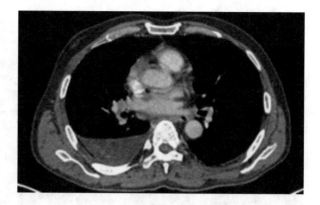

Fig. 2.4 Axial CT section—Right upper lobe is showing fibro-atelectatic patches, with tractional bronchiectatic changes

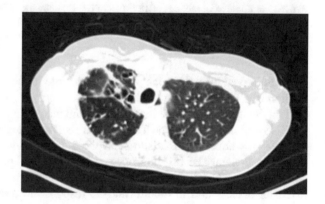

in the lung periphery and resembles a branching tree with buds at the tips of their branches. These are indicative of active tuberculosis.

Airway involvement is characterized by bronchial stenosis, leading to lobar collapse or hyperinflation, obstructive pneumonia, and mucoid impaction. Bronchial stenosis is seen in 10–40% of patients with active tuberculosis [20], which is better appreciated on CT. Pleural effusions are commoner in primary tuberculosis, but are seen in approximately 18% of patients with postprimary tuberculosis.

18F-FDG PET–CT is a molecular imaging modality, which utilizes fluorodeoxyglucose as surrogate marker. It has very high sensitivity to pick up the active inflammatory lesions, can detect infection in the lung, and may score better performance in comparison to CT alone (Fig. 2.5). Its role in therapy response monitoring and establishment of therapeutic end point have been recently ongoing.

2.1.2.3 Extrapulmonary Tuberculosis

The most frequent sites of EPTB include the lymph nodes, peritoneum, ileocecal junction, hepatosplenic, genitouriary, central nervous system (CNS), and musculoskeletal regions. In case of disseminated EPTB, multisystem involvement is common.

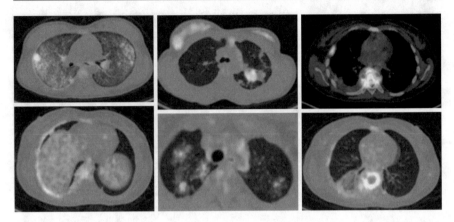

Fig. 2.5 Multiple axial sections of 18 F-FDG PET–CT showing different forms of lung involve-ment. Going clockwise from top left, extensive military nodules, consolidation in the apico-posterior segment, Pott's spine with right pleural effusion, healing consolidation, tree in bud appearance, pleural thickening

Radiological investigations play a pivotal role in the early and precise identi-fication of EPTB. Imaging modalities of choice are computed tomography (CT for lymphadenopathy and abdominal TB) and magnetic resonance imaging (MRI for CNS and musculoskeletal TB). MRI is also indicated in pediatric or pregnant patients, in whom radiation is to be avoided. In addition, bone scan may be per-formed in skeletal TB. 18F-fluorodeoxyglucose (FDG) positron emission tomog-raphy–computed tomography (PET–CT) may be used for the assessment of the extent of disease and in monitoring the response to treatment (Table 2.1). TB demonstrates a variety of clinical and radiological features depending on the organ site involved. TB can mimic a number of other disease entities, including malignancy, and it is important to be familiar with the various radiological fea-tures of TB.

2.1.3 Tuberculous Lymphadenopathy

Also called "scrofula," tuberculous lymphadenopathy is a common form of EPTB. The most commonly involved lymph nodes are cervical (~60%), followed by mediastinal (~30%), and axillary (~10%) nodes. Mostly cases present as unilat-eral cervical lymphadenopathy. With regard to features, imaging alone cannot dis-tinguish between the causes of lymphadenopathy. Biopsy has to be done for definite diagnosis. Imaging helps in guiding biopsy of these lesions (Fig. 2.6).

2.1.3.1 Ultrasonography
Matted LNDs with surrounding edema are usually seen. Doppler studies may reveal increased vascularity at the hilum. This feature helps in differentiation from malig-nant lymph nodes, which show peripheral vascularity [21].

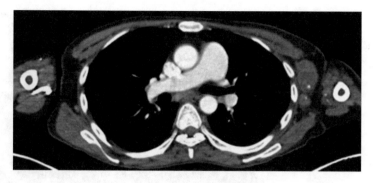

Fig. 2.6 Axial CT section—Left axillary lymphadenopathy with central hypodensity and peripheral punctate calcification

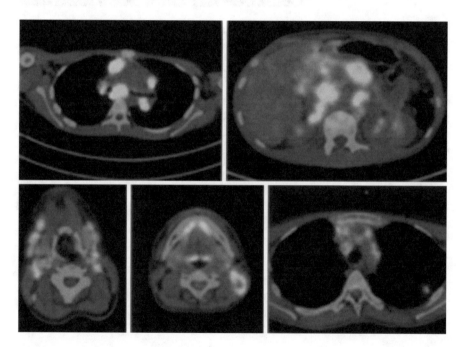

Fig. 2.7 Multiple axial sections of 18F-FDG PET–CT showing different types of lymphadenopathies. Clockwise from top left, multiple mediastinal lymphadenopathies, multiple discrete and conglomerated abdominal lymph nodes, multiple conglomerated mediastinal lymph nodes, centrally necrotic cervical lymph nodes, and multiple discrete cervical lymph nodes

2.1.3.2 CT and MRI

Multiple discrete and conglomerate enlarged lymph nodes are noted. Central areas of the necrosis are commonly seen. However, density depends on the amount of caseation, which increases with time (Fig. 2.6).

Fig. 2.8 Axial CT
section—Few hypodense
liver and splenic lesions

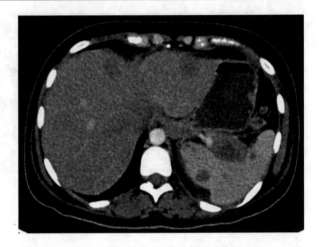

Table 2.1 Comparison of different radiological modalities for assessing tuberculosis

	CT	MRI	FDG PET–CT
Anatomical changes	Yes	Yes	Yes
Functional changes	No	No	Yes
Radiation dose to patient	Yes	No	Yes
Treatment response evaluation	Yes (size-based)	Yes (size-based)	Both anatomical and functional
Protocol followed	Regional	Regional	Whole body image in single setting
CNS TB findings	Inferior to MRI	Superior image quality	Fewer lesions detected depending on resolution or if the patient is on steroids
Musculoskeletal TB findings	Inferior to MRI	Modality of choice	Assessing disease burden and response assessment
Abdominal TB and lymphadenopathy	Modality of choice	–	Response assessment and disease burden

2.1.3.3 18F-FDG PET–CT

18F-FDG PET–CT may show peripheral uptake and central hypometabolism, depending on the amount of caseation. 18F-FDG PET–CT has the advantage of identifying all affected lymph node groups within a single setting and allows the selection of the lymph node group most suitable for biopsy (Fig. 2.7).

2.1.4   Abdominal Tuberculosis

Abdominal TB may occur directly, as in the case of primary pulmonary TB, or indirectly, via spread from the primary. It generally affects the lymph nodes, peritoneum, ileocecal junction, colon, liver, spleen, and adrenal glands. Solid organs are affected more in comparison to the gastrointestinal tract. CT is the mainstay for investigating the abdominal TB; however, knowledge of other imaging modalities, such as USG and barium enema examination, are important.

2.1.4.1 Abdominal Lymphadenopathy

Abdominal lymphadenopathy is the most common manifestation of abdominal TB, seen in 55–66% of patients [22]. On CT, the nodes are usually matted, appearing in groups, with mild peripheral fat stranding and a central necrosis, with or without calcification.

2.1.4.2 Peritoneal Tuberculosis

Peritoneal TB affects one-third of patients and is one of the most common manifestations of abdominal TB. It can be subdivided into wet, fibrotic, and dry variants [23]. On imaging, there may be significant overlap between this three. The wet type is the most common variant. It has a high protein and cellular content, which leads to high-attenuating pockets of loculated fluid or free ascites. The Hounsfield unit (HU) ranges from 20 to 45. The dry type appears as omentum caking with fibrous adhesions and mesenteric thickening. The fibrotic type presents as omental or mesenteric masses. The main imaging differential diagnoses are malignancy and peritoneal carcinomatosis [24].

2.1.4.3 Gastrointestinal Tract Tuberculosis

Due to the abundance of lymphoid tissue, the ileocecal junction (~90%) is one of the most common sites of involvement in the bowel [23]. The presentation may be ulcerative, hypertrophic, or ulcerohypertrophic forms.

Barium Studies

In the early stages, narrowing of the terminal ileum, thickening and gaping of the ileocecal valve, with thickening and hypermotility of the caecum are noted. In the chronic stages, the ileocecal valve appears relatively fixed, rigid, and incompetent, while the caecum appears shrunken in size. In the later stages, a "pulled-up" caecum may be usually noted [25]. Sometimes these lesions can lead to perforations and acute peritonitis.

Computed Tomography

Circumferential wall thickening of the terminal ileum and caecum is noted, usually in association with mesenteric lymphadenopathy. The differential diagnosis includes Crohn's disease, carcinoma, and lymphomatous involvement. Involvement of the esophagus, stomach, duodenum, and small bowel are rare.

2.1.4.4 Hepatosplenic Tuberculosis

Hepatosplenic TB presents as either miliary or macronodular involvement. The lesions are hypoattenuating on CT and may show peripheral post-contrast enhancement. The most common route of involvement is hematogenous. Macronodular involvement is less frequent and is manifested by single or multiple focal hypodense lesions, with or without peripheral rim enhancement.

On MRI, macronodular lesions appear hypointense on T1-weighted images and hyperintense on T2-weighted images, with thin peripheral and/or internal septal enhancement. The differential diagnosis includes fungal infections, sarcoidosis, lymphoma, and, rarely, metastasis [26] (Fig. 2.8).

2.1.4.5 Adrenal Tuberculosis

The adrenal glands are the most common endocrine glands involved by TB. The spread is predominantly via the hematogenous route and may be unilateral or bilateral, with central areas of caseation. When more than 90% of the cortex is involved, it may lead to primary adrenal insufficiency and a life-threatening Addisonian crisis [26].

In the early stages, smooth enlargement of the gland with low-density areas and relatively central hypo-enhancement is noted on CT [27]. In the later stages and/or in previously treated patients, gland atrophy with punctate, localized, or diffuse calcification is observed.

The MRI features are analogous to the CT appearances except for limitations when calcifications are present. 18F-FDG PET–CT shows increased metabolic activity in the adrenals in TB or any infection. Often this may be an incidental finding on PET–CT done for another diagnosis.

2.1.4.6 Genitourinary Tuberculosis

TB may involve the genitourinary tract as a secondary site following hematogenous dissemination from the lungs [28].

2.1.4.7 Renal Tuberculosis

TB at these sites accounts for 15–20% of cases of EPTB [29]. Two types are seen: pyelonephritis or a pseudo-tumor type presenting as single or multiple nodules.

The collecting system is involved in isolation or due to contiguous spread from the parenchyma. In the early stages, papillary necrosis results in caliectasis. Hydronephrosis and multifocal strictures are observed in progressive disease. Progressive hydronephrosis and parenchymal thinning with dystrophic calcification are seen in end-stage disease.

Plain radiography—On plain radiographs, foci of calcification are noted in few patients [30]. Triangular ring-like calcification in the collecting system is observed in cases of papillary necrosis. Amorphous focal ground glass-like calcification (putty kidney) is seen in end-stage disease [31].

Intravenous urography—Plain film intravenous urography is quite sensitive in detecting renal TB [32]. Many findings are observed, including parenchymal scars, moth-eaten calyces due to necrotizing papillitis, irregular caliectasis, phantom calyx, and hydronephrosis. Lower urinary tract signs include the "Kerr kink," which occurs due to abrupt narrowing at the pelviureteric junction [33].

Ultrasonography—In early-stage disease, ultrasonography may show an irregular cortical outline with few calcifications. As the disease progresses, papillary destruction with echogenic masses and distorted renal parenchyma can be observed. In end-stage disease, heavy dystrophic calcification with a small shrunken kidney is noted.

CT and MRI—CT intravenous pyelography is sensitive in identifying all manifestations of renal TB. Depending on the site of the stricture, various patterns of hydronephrosis may be seen, including focal caliectasis, caliectasis without pelvic dilatation, and generalized hydronephrosis. Other common findings include parenchymal scarring and low-attenuation parenchymal lesions. CT is also useful in depicting the extension of disease into the extrarenal space [34].

The radiological differential diagnosis of renal TB includes other causes of papillary necrosis, transitional cell carcinoma, and other infections.

2.1.5 Female Genital Organs

Involvement of the genital organs occurs in ~2% of females affected with TB. Spread may be via the hematogenous or lymphatic route. On hysterosalpingography, obstruction is usually noted at the junction of the isthmus and the ampulla [35]. A beaded appearance is seen due to multiple constrictions. A normal uterine cavity may be observed in more than 50% of cases. A further possible presentation is as an irregular filling defect with uterine synechiae and shrunken cavity. Lesions may show uptake on 18F-FDG PET–CT.

2.1.6 Male Genital Organs

Involvement of the genital organs in males is generally confined to the seminal vesicles or prostate gland, with occasional calcification. The testes and epididymites are rarely involved. Hypoattenuating lesions are noted on contrast-enhanced CT, likely representing foci of caseous necrosis. Nontuberculous pyogenic prostatic abscesses have a similar CT appearance [36]. The spread is hematogenous and self-limiting. Ultrasonography shows focal or diffuse areas of decreased echogenicity; however, these findings are nonspecific.

2.1.7 Musculoskeletal Tuberculosis

Musculoskeletal TB accounts for about 3% of all TB infections. The main route of spread is hematogenous, from lungs, or via activation of dormant infection in bone or joint post-trauma [27]. Cases of musculoskeletal TB are usually subclassified as tubercular spondylitis (50%) (also called "Potts' spine"), peripheral tuberculous arthritis (60%), osteomyelitis (38%), and soft tissue TB, including tenosynovitis and bursitis [37, 38].

2.1.7.1 Tubercular Spondylitis
The disease spread is via Batson venous plexus. The most commonly affected vertebrae are the lower thoracic and upper lumbar. The vertebral body is involved to a

greater extent than the posterior elements. The classical presentation is involvement of two or more contiguous vertebrae, with or without paravertebral abscess. In cases of anterior subligamentous involvement, the infection spreads inferiorly or superiorly without vertebral disc involvement.

Plain radiography—Potential early changes include irregular end plates and a decrease in vertebral height. Sharp angulation or gibbus deformity is noted, with anterior wedging or collapse. The displacement of paraspinal lines suggestive of psoas involvement may be noted. The calcified psoas is suggestive of an abscess.

Ultrasonography—Ultrasonography is usually helpful in identifying iliopsoas abscess and its percutaneous drainage.

CT—Cross-sectional imaging is required to better establish the extent of vertebral involvement and the possible presence of a paravertebral abscess. It presents with enhancing paravertebral soft tissue along with the vertebral involvement.

MRI—MRI is the gold standard investigation for tubercular spondylitis. MRI helps to identify the presence of an epidural component and cord compression. An early finding is focal T2 hyperintense and T1 hypointense bone marrow edema in the anterior part of vertebral body adjacent to the end plates, with heterogeneous post-contrast enhancement. Multifocal TB, compression of the spinal cord, abnormal T2 hyperintense signal in the spinal cord, and neural foraminal and neural compromise secondary to epidural collections are well demonstrated on MRI. MRI may also demonstrate the exact extent of an iliopsoas or paraspinal abscess. Small foci of involvement of posterior elements are better observed on MRI than CT [38] (Fig. 2.9).

Bone Scintigraphy
A 99mTc-methylene diphosphonate bone scan may identify multifocal sites and can sometimes be used to rule out metastasis suggested by the involvement of multiple contiguous vertebrae.

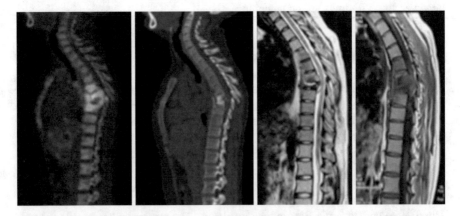

Fig. 2.9 Comparison of 18F-FDG PET–CT, CT, and T1/T2 MRI sequences in dorsal Pott's spine. Multilevel dorsal vertebral involvement with lytic destructive changes in D6, D7, and posterior displacement of the components leading to compression of the dorsal special cord

18F-FDG PET–CT

18F-FDG PET–CT may show increased uptake in tubercular spondylitis, with the identification of multiple sites, and offers further help in monitoring the response to treatment (Fig. 2.10).

2.1.8   CNS Tuberculosis

CNS TB accounts for 1% of all TB and 10–15% of EPTB. It is a leading cause of morbidity and mortality in endemic regions [39]. The spread is either hematogenous or by direct extension from local infection, such as tuberculous otomastoiditis. Manifestations of cranial TB include the following:

1. Extra-axial: Tubercular leptomeningitis and tubercular pachymeningitis
2. Intra-axial: Tuberculoma, focal cerebritis, tubercular abscess, tubercular rhomb-encephalitis, and tubercular encephalopathy.

2.1.8.1 Tubercular Leptomeningitis

Tubercular leptomeningitis (TBM) is more common than pachymeningitis. It presents with thick tuberculous exudate at the base of the brain in the subarachnoid space, predominantly in the interpeduncular fossa. Extension to the surface of the cerebral hemispheres is rare. Cerebrospinal fluid (CSF) flow may be disrupted, leading to obstructive hydrocephalus or communicating hydrocephalus due to obstruction in the basal cisterns. Ischemic infarcts due to arteritis may be seen. In addition, involvement of the second, third, fourth, and seventh cranial nerves may be observed [40].

On MRI, abnormal meningeal enhancement is noted. The magnetization transfer (MT) technique is reported to be superior in differentiating TBM from other causes of meningitis. The meninges appear hyperintense on pre-contrast T1-weighted MT

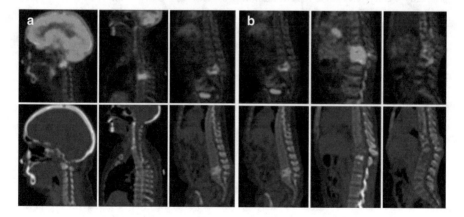

Fig. 2.10 Upper row shows 18 F-FDG PET–CT, and comparative CT section in the lower row. (**a**) Image reveals cervical, dorsal, and lumbar vertebral involvement. (**b**) Image reveals two contagious vertebrae, three contagious vertebrae, and multilevel vertebral involvement

images and enhance further on post-contrast T1-weighted MT images. The MT ratio in TBM is significantly higher than in viral meningitis, while fungal and pyogenic meningitis show a higher MT ratio compared with TBM [41].

2.1.8.2 Tubercular Pachymeningitis

Tubercular pachymeningitis is rare and is characterized by fine plaque-like regions of pachymeningeal enhancement that appear hyperdense on plain CT scan, isointense to brain on T1-weighted imaging, and isointense to hypointense on T2-weighted imaging. Homogeneous post-contrast scan enhancement is noted.

2.1.8.3 Tuberculoma

Lesions may be solitary or multiple. The most commonly affected areas are the frontal and parietal lobes. Tuberculomas may account for 15–50% of space-occupying lesions in endemic areas.

Computed Tomography

The classical presentation comprises of homogeneous ring-enhancing lesions with irregular walls of varying thickness. One-third of patients demonstrate the "target sign" (i.e., central calcification or punctate enhancement with surrounding hypoattenuation and ring enhancement) [40].

MRI

Appearances on MRI depend on whether the tuberculoma is caseating or noncaseating. Noncaseating tuberculomas are hypointense on T1-weighted and hyperintense on T2-weighted images, with homogeneous post-contrast enhancement. Caseating granulomas are isointense to hypointense on both T1- and T2-weighted images, with peripheral post-contrast enhancement. Caseating granuloma may show central T2 hyperintensity owing to liquefaction. Associated TBM may be seen. In miliary TB, tiny T2 hyperintense disc-enhancing tuberculomas are seen with TBM. They are better visualized on MT spin-echo T1-weighted images. Magnetic resonance spectroscopy is promising in the specific diagnosis of tuberculomas. A large lipid lactate peak at 1.3 ppm is characteristic, with associated reduced N-acetyl aspartate and/or slightly increased choline levels.

18F-FDG PET–CT and MRI might be complementary to each other in identifying the lesions [42].

2.1.8.4 Tubercular Abscess

Tubercular abscess accounts for 4–7% of cases in the endemic region. Presentation is as a large solitary lesion, which may be multiloculated, with surrounding vasogenic edema and mass effect. Such abscesses have pus-filled centers and vascular granulation tissue, and demonstrate an absence of epithelioid granulomatous reaction. The causative organism may be isolated from the pus, in contrast to tuberculomas.

The lesion may show vasogenic edema. Diffusion-weighted imaging reveals restricted diffusion with low apparent diffusion coefficient values. On imaging,

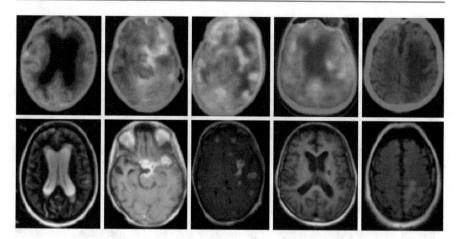

Fig. 2.11 Upper row shows 18 F-FDG PET–CT, and comparative MRI section in the lower row. Going from the left side, image reveals hydrocephalus, basal exudates, multiple central necrotic tuberculoma, tuberculosis, and vasogenic edema

pyogenic and fungal abscesses may mimic tuberculous abscess. Tuberculous abscess shows a large lipid lactate peak at 1.3 ppm on magnetic resonance spectroscopy owing to the presence of mycolic acid within the mycobacterial walls, which represents a distinguishing feature from pyogenic abscess [43] (Fig. 2.11).

2.1.8.5 Rhombencephalitis
Rhombencephalitis is a particular form of neurotuberculosis affecting the hind brain. The most common manifestation is tuberculoma.

2.1.8.6 Encephalopathy
Encephalopathy in the context of TB is most commonly observed in children and infants with pulmonary TB. The postulated mechanism is a delayed type IV hypersensitivity reaction initiated by a tuberculous protein, which leads to extensive damage of the white matter with infrequent perivascular demyelination. Imaging shows extensive unilateral or bilateral brain edema [44].

2.1.8.7 Spinal and Meningeal Involvement
Spinal TB commonly manifests as TBM and rarely as intramedullary tuberculoma. MRI is the modality of choice for the assessment of spinal TB [45]. Spinal TBM manifests as linear enhancing exudates along the spinal cord in the subarachnoid spaces and clumping of cauda equina nerve roots.

2.1.9   Other Tuberculosis

Few of the other rare tubercular sites are cardiac tuberculosis, liver tuberculosis, pancreatic tuberculosis, tubercular skin involvement, and tubercular dactylics, etc.

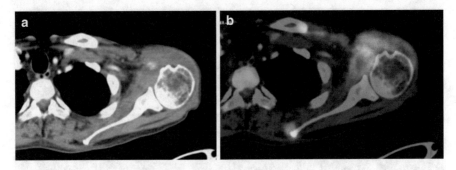

Fig. 2.12 **a** and **b** are axial CT and 18 F-FDG PET–CT sections of musculoskeletal TB, involving left shoulder joint and shoulder girdle muscles

They all have varied appearances, and imaging with HPE remains the mainstay of management (Fig. 2.12).

2.1.9.1 Emerging Role of PET–CT: Challenges and Limitations

FDG is a glucose analogue that undergoes metabolism by the same physiological processes as glucose, including being taken up by cell surface transporters (mainly the glucose transporter-1) and transformed by the rate-limiting glycolytic enzyme, hexokinase, into FDG-6-phosphate. An interesting early observation by Kubota et al. was that a substantial component of 18F-FDG uptake in tumor tissue is a result of activity localizing to peritumoral inflammatory cells, such as macrophages, which demonstrate greater 18F-FDG uptake than tumor cells. Multiple mechanistic similarities are now recognized between inflammatory and malignant cells in terms of the underlying metabolic pathways. It is this differential increase in tissue glycolysis in inflamed tissue, as opposed to normal cells, that forms the pathophysiological basis for the use of 18F-FDG PET–CT in TB.

18F-FDG PET–CT is useful in identifying the extent of disease in patients with EPTB. Tubercular lesions show high-grade metabolism, and 18F-FDG PET–CT may therefore help in selecting nodes suitable for biopsy based on metabolic uptake/standardized uptake values (SUVs). Moreover, PET–CT is more sensitive than structural imaging methods in detecting lesions.

Apart from assisting in the selection of the site for biopsy, PET–CT may play a significant role in monitoring the response to treatment. It has ability to detect changes in metabolic uptake and may have a complementary tool to anatomical imaging for this purpose [42].

2.1.9.2 TB Associated with HIV Infection

The immunocompromised status associated with HIV infection reduces the threshold for reactivation of dormant diseases such as TB. In such patients, the treatment of TB goes hand in hand with HIV treatment and can be similarly followed up with serial PET–CT scans. However, frequent monitoring is essential in these cases, as faster conversion of bacteria into resistant forms is often seen.

With the increase in extensively drug-resistant tuberculosis (XDR-TB), multidrug-resistant tuberculosis (MDR-TB), and human immunodeficiency virus (HIV) infection, an individualized therapeutic approach is gaining greater importance in this chronic inflammatory disease, which requires a sensitive diagnostic method for the assessment of not only treatment efficacy, but also initial disease spread, as well as for guidance of biopsy when equivocal findings are observed.

2.2 Conclusion

Tuberculosis has always been a crippling link in the development and prosperity of the nation, especially in the developing countries. Eradicating it from the grass-root level needs immense commitment and effective strategic planning in terms of diagnosis and treatment. For the diagnosis of TB, a physician should be aware of the role and limitations of clinical evaluation, laboratory testing, and imaging. Cross-sectional imaging plays very an important role in identifying active, inactive, and latent disease. Newer technological advancement in the diagnostic imaging and microbiological techniques will assist in early diagnosis and follow-up of the patients.

References

1. Kochi A. The global tuberculosis situation and the new control strategy of the World Health Organization. Tubercle. 1991;72(1):1–6.
2. World Health Organization. WHO Global Tuberculosis Report 2016. WHO, 2018. Available online: http://www.who.int/tb/publications/global_report/en.
3. Pai M, Denkinger CM, Kik SV, Rangaka MX, Zwerling A, Oxlade O, et al. Gamma interferon release assays for detection of Mycobacterium tuberculosis infection. Clin Microbiol Rev. 2014;27(1):3–20.
4. Siddiqi K. Clinical diagnosis of smear-negative pulmonary tuberculosis in low-income countries: the current evidence. Lancet Infect Dis. 2003;3:288.
5. Steingart KR, Henry M, Ng V, Hopewell PC, Ramsay A, Cunningham J, et al. Fluorescence versus conventional sputum smear microscopy for tuberculosis: a systematic review. Lancet Infect Dis. 2006;6(9):570–81.
6. Tapley A, Switz N, Reber C, Davis JL, Miller C, Matovu JB, et al. Mobile digital fluorescence microscopy for diagnosis of tuberculosis. J Clin Microbiol. 2013;51(6):1774–8.
7. Cruciani M, Scarparo C, Malena M, Bosco O, Serpelloni G, Mengoli C. Meta-analysis of BACTEC MGIT 960 and BACTEC 460 TB, with or without solid media, for detection of mycobacteria. J Clin Microbiol. 2004;42(5):2321–5.
8. World Health Organization. Use of liquid TB culture and drug susceptibility testing (DST) in low- and medium-income settings. Geneva: World Health Organization; 2007.
9. Ling DI, Zwerling AA, Pai M. GenoType MTBDR assays for the diagnosis of multidrug-resistant tuberculosis: a meta-analysis. Eur Respir J. 2008;32(5):1165–74.
10. Steingart KR, Sohn H, Schiller I, et al. Xpert® MTB/RIF assay for pulmonary tuberculosis and rifampicin resistance in adults. Cochrane Database Syst Rev. 2013;(1):CD009593.

11. Minion J, Leung E, Menzies D, Pai M. Microscopic-observation drug susceptibility and thin layer agar assays for the detection of drug resistant tuberculosis: a systematic review and meta-analysis. Lancet Infect Dis. 2010;10(10):688–98.
12. Marais BJ, Pai M. New approaches and emerging technologies in the diagnosis of childhood tuberculosis. Paediatr Respir Rev. 2007;8(2):124–33.
13. Steingart KR, Flores LL, Dendukuri N, Schiller I, Laal S, Ramsay A, et al. Commercial serological tests for the diagnosis of active pulmonary and extrapulmonary tuberculosis: an updated systematic review and meta-analysis. PLoS Med. 2011;8(8):e1001062.
14. Minion J, Leung E, Talbot E, Dheda K, Pai M, Menzies D. Diagnosing tuberculosis with urine lipoarabinomannan: systematic review and meta-analysis. Eur Respir J. 2011;38(6):1398–405.
15. Andreu J, Caceres J, Pallisa E, Martinez-Rodriguez M. Radiological manifestations of pulmonary tuberculosis. Eur J Radiol. 2004;51(2):139–49.
16. World Health Organization. Tuberculosis prevalence surveys: a handbook. 2011.
17. Cruz R. Digital radiography, image archiving and image display: practical tips. Can Vet J. 2008;49(11):1122.
18. Curvo-Semedo L, Teixeira L, Caseiro-Alves F. Tuberculosis of the chest. Eur J Radiol. 2005;55(2):158–72.
19. Woodring JH, Vandiviere HM, Fried AM, Dillon ML, Williams TD, Melvin IG. Update: the radio-graphic features of pulmonary tuberculosis. AJR Am J Roentgenol. 1986;146(3):497–506.
20. McAdams HP, Erasmus J, Winter JA. Radiological manifestations of pulmonary tuberculosis. Radiol Clin N Am. 1995;33(4):655–78.
21. Ahuja A, Ying M, Yuen YH, Metreweli C. Power Doppler sonography to differentiate tuberculous cervical lymphadenopathy from nasopharyngeal carcinoma. AJNR Am J Neuroradiol. 2001;22:735–40.
22. Leder RA, Low VH. Tuberculosis of the abdomen. Radiol Clin N Am. 1995;33:691–705.
23. Suri S, Gupta S, Suri R. Computed tomography in abdominal tuberculosis. Br J Radiol. 1999;72:92–8.
24. Takalkar AM, Bruno GL, Reddy M, Lilien DL. Intense FDG activity in peritoneal tuberculosis mimics peritoneal carcinomatosis. Clin Nucl Med. 2007;32:244–6.
25. Nakano H, Jaramillo E, Watanabe M, Miyachi I, Takahama K, Itoh M. Intestinal tuberculosis: findings on double contrast barium enema. Gastrointest Radiol. 1992;17:108–14.
26. Huang YC, Tang YL, Zhang XM, Zeng NL, Li R, Chen TW. Evaluation of primary adrenal insufficiency secondary to tuberculosis adrenalitis with computed tomography and magnetic resonance imaging: current status. World J Radiol. 2015;7:336–42.
27. Buxi TB, Vohra RB, Sujatha, Byotra SP, Mukherji S, Daniel M. CT enlargement due to tuberculosis: a review of literature with five new cases. Clin Imaging. 1992;16:102–8.
28. Pasternak MS, Rubin RH. Urinary tract tuberculosis. In: Schrier RW, editor. Diseases of the kidney and urinary tract. 7th ed. Philadelphia, PA: Lippincott Williams & Wilkins; 2001. p. 1017–37.
29. Burrill J, Williams CJ, Bain G, Conder G, Hine AL, Misra RR. Tuberculosis: a radiologic review. Radiographics. 2007;27:1255–73.
30. Kollins SA, Hartman GW, Carr DT, Segura JW, Hattery RR. Roentgenographic findings in urinary tract tuberculosis: a 10 year review. Am J Roentgenol Radium Therapy, Nucl Med. 1974;121:487–99.
31. Davidson AJ, Hartman DS, Choyke PL, Wagner BJ. Parenchymal disease with normal size and contour. In: Davidson AJ, editor. Davidson's radiology of the kidney and genitourinary tract. 3rd ed. Philadelphia, PA: Saunders; 1999. p. 327–58.
32. Kenney PJ. Imaging of chronic renal infections. AJR Am J Roentgenol. 1990;155:485–94.
33. Berry M. Diagnostic radiology, urogenital imaging. New Delhi: Jaypee Brothers Publishers; 2003.
34. Wang LJ, Wong YC, Chen CJ, Lim KE. CT features of genitourinary tuberculosis. J Comput Assist Tomogr. 1997;21:254–8.
35. Jung YY, Kim JK, Cho KS. Genitourinary tuberculosis: comprehensive cross-sectional imaging. AJR Am J Roentgenol. 2005;184:143–50.

36. Harisinghani MG, McLoud TC, Shepard JA, Ko JP, Shroff MM, Mueller PR. Tuberculosis from head to toe. Radiographics. 2000;20:449–70.
37. Jaovisidha S, Chen C, Ryu KN, et al. Tuberculous tenosynovitis and bursitis: imaging findings in 21 cases. Radiology. 1996;201(2):507–13.
38. Martini M, Adjrad A, Boudjemaa A. Tuberculous osteomyelitis: a review of 125 cases. Int Orthop. 1986;10:201–7.
39. Garg RK. Classic diseases revisited: tuberculosis of the central nervous system. Postgrad Med J. 1999;75:133–40.
40. Morgado C, Ruivo N. Imaging meningo-encephalic tuberculosis. Eur J Radiol. 2005;55:188–92.
41. Gupta RK, Kathuria MK, Pradhan S. Magnetization transfer MR imaging in CNS tuberculosis. AJNR Am J Neuroradiol. 1999;20:867–75.
42. Gambhir S, Kumar M, Ravina M, Bhoi SK, Kalita J, Misra UK. Role of 18F-FDG PET in demonstrating disease burden in patients with tuberculous meningitis. J Neurol Sci. 2016;370:196–200.
43. Luthra G, Parihar A, Nath K, Jaiswal S, Prasad KN, Husain N, et al. Comparative evaluation of fungal, tubercular, and pyogenic brain abscesses with conventional and diffusion MR imaging and proton MR spectroscopy. AJNR Am J Neuroradiol. 2007;28:1332.
44. Patkar D, Narang J, Yanamandala R, Lawande M, Shah GV. Central nervous system tuberculosis: pathophysiology and imaging findings. Neuroimaging Clin N Am. 2012;22:677–705.
45. Sinan T, Al-Khawari H, Ismail M, Ben-Nakhi A, Sheikh Spinal M. Tuberculosis: CT and MRI feature. Ann Saudi Med. 2004;24:437–41.

Radiological Imaging in Tuberculosis

3

Ruza Stevic and Strahinja Odalovic

Contents

R. Stevic (✉)
Faculty of Medicine, University of Belgrade, Belgrade, Serbia

Center for Radiology and Magnetic Resonance, Clinical Center of Serbia, Belgrade, Serbia

S. Odalovic
Faculty of Medicine, University of Belgrade, Belgrade, Serbia

Center for Nuclear Medicine, Clinical Center of Serbia, Belgrade, Serbia

© Springer Nature Switzerland AG 2020
D. Sobic Saranovic et al. (eds.), *PET/CT in Tuberculosis*, Clinicians' Guides to
Radionuclide Hybrid Imaging, https://doi.org/10.1007/978-3-030-47009-8_3

Chest radiographs play the most important role in the screening, diagnosis, and response to the treatment of patients with tuberculosis (TB). However, non-specificity of findings, failure to detect hilar and mediastinal lymphadenopathy, and overlooking of subtle parenchymal abnormalities have made this method obsolete. Computerized tomography (CT) nowadays represents standard imaging modality in detection of active pulmonary tuberculosis [1].

3.1   Primary Pulmonary Tuberculosis

The manifestations of primary pulmonary tuberculosis include gangliopulmonary TB (airspace consolidation and lymphadenopathy), pleural effusion, miliary disease, and tracheobronchial TB. Only the gangliopulmonary form is characteristic of primary TB and other manifestations may be seen in postprimary disease as well [2].

Lymphadenopathy is one of the most common radiological signs of primary tuberculosis. CT is more sensitive in detection of enlarged lymph nodes compared to chest X-ray. The lymphadenopathy is usually unilateral, and the most common affected sites are hilum and paratracheal region [2]. Bilateral lymphadenopathy is observed in about one-third of patients with primary TB. Contrast-enhanced CT of enlarged lymph nodes shows low-attenuation centers corresponding to caseous necrosis and peripheral rim opacification [3] (Fig. 3.1a). Associated parenchymal consolidations are on the same site as enlarged lymph nodes in up to two-thirds of pediatric patients with primary TB. On CT, parenchymal consolidation is most commonly dense and homogeneous, usually located in lower lung lobes, without side or lobar predilection. The air bronchogram may be seen. Patchy, nodular, or linear infiltrates are less common [2, 3] (Fig. 3.1b). Cavitations are rare, occurring mainly with progression of the disease [3]. Usually, primary tuberculosis is self-limiting

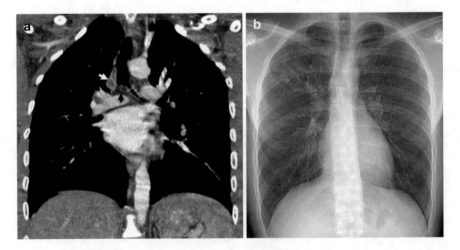

Fig. 3.1 Gangliopulmonary TB: (**a**) CT (coronal view) shows right paratracheal and subcarinal lymph nodes with low-attenuation centers and rim postcontrast opacification (arrows). (**b**) Chest radiography of the same patients show patchy infiltrates in the right upper lobe

disease in immunocompetent patients. The resolution of primary tuberculosis consolidation is usually slow, and residual calcified scar and fibrotic changes may remain, such as Ghon tubercle which together with calcified hilar or mediastinal lymph nodes constitute Ranke complex [3–5].

Complications of gangliopulmonary TB include perforation of an enlarged LN into a bronchus, bronchial compression due to adenopathy causing retro-obstructive pneumonia, and/or atelectasis [1].

3.2 Postprimary Pulmonary Tuberculosis

Postprimary pulmonary tuberculosis (secondary or reactivation tuberculosis) usually occurs in adults and adolescents who have developed immunity to primary tuberculosis infection [6]. It presents the either endogenous reactivation of latent infection with dormant bacilli in residual foci or reinfection with *M. tuberculosis* [7]. The presentation of disease and radiological features largely depend on immune status of the host. Although the radiological appearance of primary and postprimary tuberculosis is thought to be quite distinct, recent DNA fingerprinting studies showed similarity in radiological manifestations of both clinical entities [8, 9].

Early radiological features of postprimary tuberculosis include inhomogeneous or patchy consolidation in upper lung areas [10]. This form of disease has high predilection for apical and posterior segments of upper lobes, and superior segments of lower lobes [5, 10]. In the majority of cases, more than one segment is affected, with bilateral disease in up to two-thirds of patients [11]. The liquefaction of caseous necrosis is the following event, with subsequent communication with tracheobronchial tree and formation of cavities [4]. Cavities are the hallmark of postprimary tuberculosis and occur in around 50% of patients during the course of the disease, and they are frequently multiple and may vary in size [10–12]. In early, active phase of the disease cavitations have thick, irregular walls, which become thin and smooth during healing process (Fig. 3.2). Ultimately, cavitation may progress to

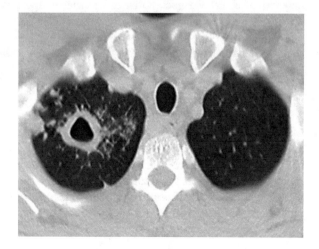

Fig. 3.2 Axial CT of thick-walled cavity in right upper lobe in patient with postprimary TB

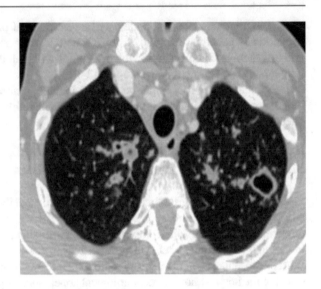

Fig. 3.3 Bronchogenic spread: Axial CT demonstrates thick-walled cavity in left upper lobe and scattered small nodules

emphysematous bullae, without fibrotic scar [10]. Air–fluid level in cavity is manifestation of superimposed bacterial or fungal infestation. Cavities may communicate with pleura, resulting in pleurisy and empyema, or with blood vessels, leading to hematogenous dissemination or hemoptysis [4].

Bronchogenic spread of tuberculous pathogens is the most common way of dissemination from cavities, when active tuberculosis communicates with bronchial tree [3, 10]. This form of the disease is radiographically detected in around one-fifth of cases [13]. Chest radiography is insensitive for these morphological changes. CT reveals small ill-defined nodules (2–4 mm in diameter) disseminated throughout both lungs, with centrilobular distribution, usually affecting lower lung areas [4, 13] (Fig. 3.3). A significant radiologic finding on CT is the "tree-in-bud" pattern, consisting of multiple branching linear structures representing caseation necrosis in the respiratory and terminal bronchioles [5, 13] (Fig. 3.4). However, these radiological features may involve apical and apico-posterior segments of upper lung lobes as well [8].

3.3   Radiological Patterns Encountered in Both Primary and/or Postprimary TB

3.3.1   Miliary Tuberculosis

Miliary tuberculosis presents hematogenous spread of the TB, suggesting progressive disease with bad prognosis and high mortality rate [3]. This form of the disease can be a manifestation of both primary and postprimary disease, but is more common in the primary form, and rarely in the setting of the postprimary disease [4]. It is characterized with diffuse micronodular changes in lung parenchyma. Miliary tuberculosis is very difficult to detect on plain chest radiography. CT shows

Fig. 3.4 Bronchogenic spread: Axial CT displays branching and nodular opacities ("tree-in-bud" pattern) in right upper lobe

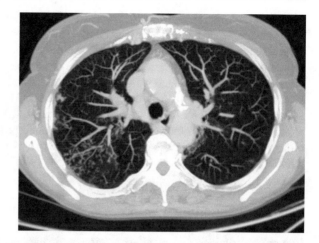

Fig. 3.5 Miliary TB: Axial CT scan shows innumerable 1–3 mm nodules with random distribution throughout both lungs, with a sign of coalescence in the left upper lobe

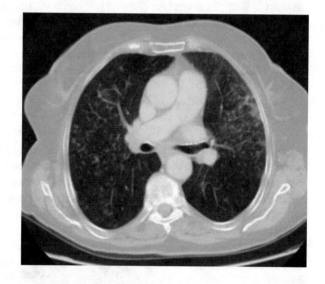

micronodules, randomly distributed around small blood vessels, measuring 1–3 mm in diameter (Fig. 3.5). These nodules may conflate creating the "snowstorm" image [2–5].

3.3.2 Pleural Tuberculosis

Pleural effusions are common manifestations of active primary disease, and are usually unilateral [5]. Also, pleural involvement may complicate postprimary TB. In postprimary TB, pleural effusions are almost always the result of pleural communication with cavity, and therefore effusion samples may be positive to the presence of *M. tuberculosis* [4]. During the early stage, there is free pleural effusion between smoothly thickened parietal and visceral pleura. Contrast-enhanced CT shows split pleura sign [5]. In fibro-purulent phase, the effusion is denser, with septations, sometimes consisting only pus, suggesting the presence of empyema. In this phase, effusion may be complicated with bronchopleural fistula, manifested with air–fluid level, or cutaneous extension—empyema necessitatis [3]. Long-standing empyema after resolution may result in chronic fluid collections, with thickened and calcified pleura (Fig. 3.6). Fibrothorax, as the result of healing process, is manifested with diffuse pleural thickening, calcifications, and loss of volume of hemithorax, but without effusion [4].

3.3.3   Tracheobronchial TB

Primary tuberculosis can manifest as airway disease, but this form is much more frequent in postprimary tuberculosis [3]. When it occurs, bronchial stenosis due to either direct endobronchial spread or extrinsic compression from enlarged lymph nodes is demonstrated. Radiography features include indirect signs, such as atelectasis, postobstructive pneumonia, or hyperinflation. Sometimes, endobronchial narrowing with irregular wall thickening can be seen on CT [3, 5].

3.4   Complications

Pulmonary tuberculosis is associated with various complications, and their prevalence increases with the duration of the disease. These complications include bronchiectasis, pulmonary aspergillosis, airway stenosis, tuberculoma, chronic obstructive pulmonary disease, lung destruction, scar carcinoma, fistulae formation, and vascular complications (pseudoaneurysms, hypertrophied bronchial arteries, and systemic collaterals) [14].

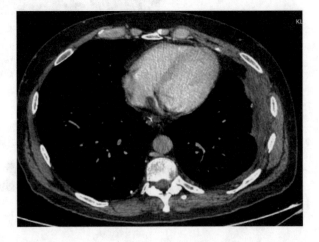

Fig. 3.6 Tuberculous pleuritis: Axial CT scan shows a left-sided encapsulated pleural effusion with marked pleural thickening

Fig. 3.7 Bronchiectasis: Axial CT scan shows dilatation of bronchi within middle lobe

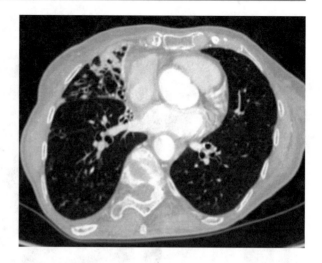

The bronchiectasis, resulting from scaring of lung parenchyma and retraction of hila are more common in upper lung area in patients with postprimary TB. These are usually traction bronchiectasis which present on chest radiography or CT as small cystic or ring-like opacities, which may present with air–fluid level or as round opacities in cases of superinfection [5] (Fig. 3.7).

Aspergillosis, infection with aspergillus fumigatus, is a common complication of pulmonary tuberculosis. It is manifested as noninvasive mycetoma/aspergilloma [14]. The characteristic radiographic feature of aspergilloma is thin ring-like shadow, representing tuberculous cavity, with round mass-like opacity within the ring in gravity-dependent position, with air crescent sign [5] (Fig. 3.8).

3.5 Extrapulmonary Tuberculosis

Although tuberculosis is mostly limited to the lung, occasionally it may have an extrathoracic spread and involve various organs. This is often the case in immuno-compromised patients, in whom genitourinary system, musculoskeletal system, and/or central nervous system may be affected [15].

3.5.1 Genitourinary Tuberculosis

The genitourinary tract is the most common site of extrathoracic TB infection after hematogenous dissemination, contributing to 14–41% of all extrathoracic TB infections [16]. The intravenous urography (IVU) is very sensitive in detection of TB. The earliest sign is minimal dilation of calyces, followed by irregularity of calyceal margin, and ultimately showing the moth-eaten appearance [15, 16]. Later, during the course of disease, extensive cavitation, cortical scars,

Fig. 3.8 Aspergilloma: Coronal view CT demonstrates thin-walled cavities in both upper lobes colonized by an aspergilloma

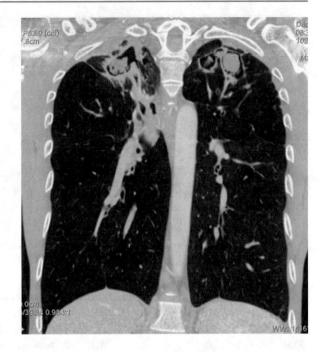

masses, calcifications, and perinephric abscesses are formed [16, 17]. However, lesions that are more prone for renal function damage include strictures of collecting tract, especially strictures of lower ureter, ureteropelvic junction, and neck of the calyx, resulting in regional caliectasis and hydronephrosis. In these cases, hydronephrosis is a commonly irregularity marginated with filling defect due to caseous debris [16, 18]. Urinary bladder manifestations of TB infection include wall thickening, ulcerations, and filling defect caused by granulomatous material. Salpingitis with obstruction and dilatation may be observed in women with TB, while calcified lesions and hypodense lesions may be observed in TB infection of prostate in men [15].

3.5.2 Musculoskeletal Tuberculosis

Musculoskeletal TB occurs in 1–3% of TB patients, with tuberculous spondylitis being the most common manifestation [19]. Radiographic features of early-stage TB spondylitis include radiolucencies and loss of definition of end-plates [20]. This is followed by vertebral collapse and anterior wedging, causing kyphosis and gibbus deformity [15]. CT enables better lesion characterization and evaluation of its extent [21]. MR imaging is accurate for differentiation of tuberculous from pyogenic spondylitis. Paraspinal masses and abscesses develop in early stage, localized anterolateral to the spine, displacing anterior longitudinal ligament, almost exclusively associated with vertebral infection (Fig. 3.9a, b). Paraspinal abscess formation are

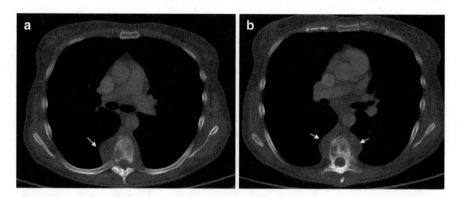

Fig. 3.9 (**a, b**) Tuberculous spondylitis: Axial CT scans of dorsal spine show multilevel fragmentary bone patterns and paraspinal soft tissue abscesses (arrows)

usually localized in thoracic spine, with extension through the iliopsoas compartment, occasionally reaching retroperitoneum, pelvis, or even thighs [20]. On CT they are hypodense with rim postcontrast opacification [21].

The less frequent musculoskeletal manifestations of TB include arthritis, osteomyelitis, tenosynovitis, and bursitis. TB arthritis is a result of hematogenous dissemination, which rarely occurs after direct intraarticular spread from adjacent bone lesions. Transphyseal spread is specific for TB, and very unusual in pyogenic infections [19]. TB arthritis is usually monoarticular, with hip and knee being the most common locations, and radiographic features include periarticular osteoporosis, peripheral bone erosion, and narrowing of joint space—Phemister's triad [19].

3.5.3   Central Nervous System Tuberculosis

The involvement of central nervous system (CNS) is present in about 5% of TB patients. The most common manifestation is tuberculous meningitis, with parenchymal lesions, such as tuberculomas, tuberculous abscesses, and miliary TB being less common [15]. Tuberculous meningitis usually is a result of hematogenous spread of *M. tuberculosis*. The most common finding of TB meningitis on CT is isodense or slightly hyperdense exudate which obliterates basal cisterns [22]. This entity is better evaluated on MR [23]. Tuberculomas, as the most common parenchymal lesions in CNS, may be solitary or multiple. On nonenhanced CT images, these lesions are isodense or hyperdense, with ring-like opacification on contrast-enhanced CT. Target sign, consisting of central calcification surrounded with ring-like opacification, is quite specific [22]. Tuberculous abscesses are a rare TB complication, characterized with central hypodense area of liquefaction, with surrounding edema and mass effect [22]. Miliary tuberculosis of CNS is manifested with multiple small tubercles (<2 mm), occasionally seen on MR as high intensity foci on T2 or small enhanced lesions on postcontrast T1 [24].

3.5.4   Gastrointestinal Tuberculosis

Gastrointestinal tract is not commonly involved in tuberculosis infection. Esophageal involvement is very rare, usually as a part of secondary manifestation of tuberculosis reactivation [25, 26]. Barium enema shows extrinsic compression (due to enlarged lymph nodes), strictures, diverticula, and fistulae. CT reveals eccentric wall thickening and tumor-like masses, accompanied with lymphadenopathy and lung changes suggestive of TB infection [27] (Fig. 3.10). Abdominal TB is usually manifested as lymphadenopathy, with enlarged retroperitoneal and mesenterial lymph nodes. Concentric mural thickening of ileocecal junction is by far the most common gastrointestinal TB manifestation [15]. Like the other gastrointestinal TB manifestations, primary liver tuberculosis is not common, but it may be associated with pulmonary or miliary TB. However, neither clinical presentation nor imaging features of hepatic TB involvement are specific. Tuberculous focus in the liver is usually manifested as hypodense lesion with peripheral postcontrast enhancement in portal phase, thus mimicking hepatic cholangiocellular carcinoma. The diagnosis of TB can be assumed if other clinical signs of TB infection are present, together with imaging findings of pulmonary or miliary TB [28]. Pancreas tuberculosis is extremely rare, with wide range of image findings which are highly nonspecific. CT features include hypodense mass with irregular margins and rim postcontrast opacification or cystic lesions with multilocular appearance, associated with low-density peripancreatic lymph nodes [29].

Extrapulmonary manifestation of TB infection may also include cardiac involvement, with tuberculous pericarditis being the most common pathology as well as cutaneous dissemination (scrofuloderma). Other TB extrathoracic manifestations are extremely rare [15].

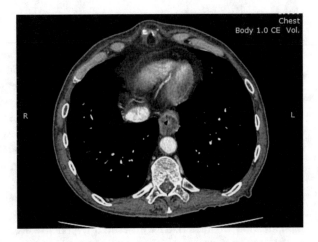

Fig. 3.10 Axial CT demonstrates eccentric wall-thickening of the mid-portion of esophagus in patient with pulmonary TB reactivation

References

1. Jeong YJ, Lee KS. Pulmonary tuberculosis: up-to-date imaging and management. AJR. 2008;191:834–44.
2. Bomanji JB, Gupta N, Gulati P, Das CJ. Imaging in tuberculosis. Cold Spring Harb Perspect Med. 2015;5:a017814.
3. Nachiappan AC, Rahbar K, Shi X, Guy ES, Mortani Barbosa EJ Jr, Shroff GS, et al. Pulmonary tuberculosis: role of radiology in diagnosis and management. Radiographics. 2017;37:52–72.
4. Bhalla AS, Goyal A, Guleria R, Gupta AK. Chest tuberculosis: radiological review and imaging recommendations. Indian J Radiol Imaging. 2015;25:213–25.
5. McLoud TC, Boiselle PM. Pulmonary infections in the normal host. In: McLoud TC, Boiselle PM, editors. Thoracic radiology: the requisites. 2nd ed. Philadelphia, PA: Mosby Elsevier; 2010. p. 80–120.
6. Hunter RL. The pathogenesis of tuberculosis: the early infiltrate of post-primary (adult pulmonary) tuberculosis: a distinct disease entity. Front Immunol. 2018;9:2108.
7. Rook GAW, Bchir MB. The immunology and pathogenesis of tuberculosis. In: Madkour MM, editor. Tuberculosis. Berlin Heidelberg: Springer-Verlag; 2004. p. 133–51.
8. Yoon JY, Lee IJ, Im HJ, Lee K, Lee Y, Bae SH. CT findings in apical versus basal involvement of pulmonary tuberculosis. Diagn Interv Radiol. 2013;19:85–90.
9. Marais BJ, Parker SK, Verver S, van Rie A, Warren RM. Primary and Postprimary or reactivation tuberculosis: time to revise confusing terminology? Am J Roentgenol. 2009;192:W198.
10. Curvo-Semedo L, Teixcira L, Caseiro-Alves F. Tuberculosis of the chest. Eur J Radiol. 2005;55:158–72.
11. Burrill J, Williams CJ, Bain G, Conder G, Hine AL, Misra RR. Tuberculosis: a radiologic review. Radiographics. 2007;27:1255–73.
12. Gadkowski LB, Stout JE. Cavitary pulmonary disease. Clin Microbiol Rev. 2008;21:305–33.
13. Fujita J, Bandoh S, Kubo A, Ishii T, Kanaji N, Nakamura H, et al. HRCT shows variations in appearance in disseminated tuberculosis in adults. Int J Tuberc Lung Dis. 2006;10:222–6.
14. Chakaya J, Kirenga B, Getahun H. Long term complications after completion of pulmonary tuberculosis treatment: a quest for a public health approach. J Clin Tuberc Mycobact Dis. 2016;3:10–2.
15. Maclean KA, Becker AK, Chang SD, Harris AC. Extrapulmonary tuberculosis: imaging features beyond the chest. Can Assoc Radiol J. 2013;64:319–24.
16. Merchant S, Bharati A, Merchant N. Tuberculosis of the genitourinary system - urinary tract tuberculosis: renal tuberculosis—part I. Indian J Radiol Imaging. 2013;23:46–63.
17. Zagoria RJ. Renal masses. In: Zagoria RJ, Dyer R, Brady C, editors. Genitourinary imaging: the requisites. 3rd ed. Philadelphia, PA: Elsevier; 2016. p. 66–106.
18. Zagoria RJ. The renal synus, pelvicocaliceal system, and ureter. In: Zagoria RJ, Dyer R, Brady C, editors. Genitourinary imaging: the requisites. 3rd ed. Philadelphia, PA: Elsevier; 2016. p. 146–89.
19. De Backer AI, Vanhoenacker FM, Sanghvi DA. Imaging features of extraaxial musculoskeletal tuberculosis. Indian J Radiol Imaging. 2009;19:176–86.
20. Rivas-Garcia A, Sarria-Estrada S, Torrents-Odin C, Casas-Gomila L, Franquet E. Imaging findings of Pott's disease. Eur Spine J. 2013;22(Suppl 4):567–78.
21. Jung NY, Jee WH, Ha KY, Park CK, Byun JY. Discrimination of tuberculous spondylitis from pyogenic spondylitis on MRI. AJR. 2004;182:1405–10.
22. Taheri MS, Karimi MA, Haghighatkhah H, Pourghorban R, Samadian M, Kasmaei HD. Central nervous system tuberculosis: an imaging-focused review of a Reemerging disease. Radiol Res Pract. 2015;2015:202806.
23. Parmar H, Sitoh YY, Anand P, Chua V, Hui F. Contrast-enhanced flair imaging in the evaluation of infectious leptomeningeal diseases. Eur J Radiol. 2006;58:89–95.

24. Trivedi R, Saksena S, Gupta RK. Magnetic resonance imaging in central nervous system tuberculosis. Indian J Radiol Imaging. 2009;19:256–65.
25. Gomes J, Antunes A, Carvalho A, Duarte R. Dysphagia as a manifestation of esophageal tuberculosis: a report of two cases. J Med Case Rep. 2011;5:447. https://doi.org/10.1186/1752-1947-5-447.
26. Jain SK, Jain S, Jain M, Yaduvanshi A. Esophageal tuberculosis: is it so rare? Report of 12 cases and review of the literature. Am J Gastroenterol. 2002;97:287–91.
27. Nagi B, Lal A, Kochhar R, Bhasin DK, Gulati M, Suri S, et al. Imaging of esophageal tuberculosis: a review of 23 cases. Acta Radiol. 2003;44:329–33.
28. Park JI. Primary hepatic tuberculosis mimicking intrahepatic cholangiocarcinoma: report of two cases. Ann Surg Treat Res. 2015;89:98–101.
29. Chaudhary P, Bhadana U, Arora MP. Pancreatic tuberculosis. Indian J Surg. 2015;77:517–24.

Management of Tuberculosis

4

A. O. Ankrah

Contents

A. O. Ankrah (✉)
Department of Nuclear Medicine, Steve Biko Academic Hospital, University of Pretoria, Pretoria, South Africa

Department of Nuclear Medicine and Molecular Imaging, University Medical Center Groningen, University of Groningen, Groningen, Netherlands

National Centre for Radiotherapy and Nuclear Medicine, Korle Bu Teaching Hospital, Accra, Ghana

© Springer Nature Switzerland AG 2020
D. Sobic Saranovic et al. (eds.), *PET/CT in Tuberculosis*, Clinicians' Guides to Radionuclide Hybrid Imaging, https://doi.org/10.1007/978-3-030-47009-8_4

4.1   Introduction

Tuberculosis (TB) is a public health hazard of pandemic proportions. The development of drug resistance and the HIV pandemic has made the management of tuberculosis even more complicated. The management of TB requires the involvement of multiple disciplines and various sectors of society. There is a need for political buy-in at the highest level of government as the TB pandemic cannot be ended without social interventions such as poverty alleviation, improved healthcare, and building or restructuring of facilities where TB transmission is known to be high, such as in hospitals or prisons. There is also the need to invest heavily in drug-development research as resistance to TB drugs is an ever-present problem and vaccines are not efficient at preventing transmission. The significant decrease in the prevalence and incidence of TB in developed countries to the current low level is evidence of how improvement in socioeconomic circumstances may reduce TB prevalence and incidence. TB can be easily spread from one country to another via air travel, which makes it imperative for all countries to join in the fight against TB. There is a concerted effort from all nations of the world through the World Health Organization (WHO) and the United Nations (UN) to end the TB epidemic by 2030 [1, 2].

The management of the infection includes the following:

4.2   Prevention

4.2.1   Individuals

- Vaccination
- Treatment of people with latent TB who are likely to progress to active disease (here novel tools such as positron emission tomography (PET)/computed tomography (CT) imaging may play an important role in identifying such individuals)
- Personal respiratory hygiene as part of infection control measure
  TB Infection control—especially in healthcare facilities and other densely populated settings—requires the following measures:
- Administrative
- Environmental
- Personal respiratory hygiene

4.2.2   Community

- Community participation to increase awareness and reduce stigmatization
- Improvement of socioeconomic status (poverty drives TB through malnutrition, overcrowding, and alcoholism)

4.2.3 International

- In low-burden countries, there is a need for screening and treatment of people with active disease

4.3 Treatment of Active Disease

- TB drugs (for both drug-susceptible and drug-resistant disease)
- Surgical intervention in selected cases

4.4 Management of Comorbid Conditions

- Antiretroviral therapy for patients with HIV
- Universal health coverage, including treatment of conditions that allow TB to flourish such as diabetes mellitus

4.5 Vaccination

Bacilli Calmette–Guérin (BCG) is the current vaccine against TB in children. BCG is useful in reducing the incidence of disseminated TB and TB meningitis in children. The vaccine is not as effective in reducing the progression from latent to active TB infection in adults. The use of BCG in national childhood immunization programs of countries depends on the epidemiology of TB in the country. In 2017, 158 countries offered childhood BCG immunization, with 120 reporting at least 90% coverage. Researchers are actively looking for a vaccine that would either prevent infection or prevent the progression of latent infection to active disease [1].

4.6 Treatment of Patients with Latent TB Who Are Likely to Progress to Active Disease

TB prevention of latent infection progressing to active disease requires isoniazid, rifampicin, or rifapentine. Rifampicin is administered as a daily dose for 4 months for prevention of TB. Isoniazid can be used in different doses as a single agent daily for 9 months or twice weekly (in a higher dose) for 9 months. A 6-month daily dose or a twice-weekly dose of isoniazid is also available. A combination of rifapentine and isoniazid as a weekly dose for 3 months is used to prevent active TB in patients with latent infection. As a result of the new recommendation introduced by the WHO in 2018, the number of patients who need preventive therapy has expanded, and the proportion of such patients accessing health care is relatively low [3–5].

Identification of such individuals with a high risk of progressing to active disease may in future be possible with novel PET imaging possibilities.

4.7   TB Infection Control

Infection control is essential for health facilities and other places with large congregations of people where the risk of TB transmission is high. In high TB burden countries particularly, early identification of TB cases and isolation are considered the most important means of infection prevention in health facilities. An infection control policy for TB should ideally be part of the general infection control policy. There should be policies in place at various levels on identifying suspected TB cases, on collection of sputum samples, and on handling of samples in the laboratory. Contact time between healthcare workers and infected patients should be kept to a minimum. Where possible, most patients should be managed on an outpatient basis in the absence of comorbid conditions. Patients should be educated on infection control measures such as reduced contact with children and sleeping alone if possible, among others. For environmental control, natural ventilation should be maximized, and direction of airflow should be controlled where weather conditions allow. In environments where the weather does not allow, systems that exchange the air may be deployed if such resources are available. Health personnel should wear appropriate-sized masks when available and should be aware that the normal surgical mask does not protect against TB [6, 7].

4.8   Drug Treatment of Active TB

The appropriate treatment of TB depends on whether the TB strain is drug-susceptible or drug-resistant as determined by drug susceptibility testing. As the results of such drug susceptibility tests may take weeks to become available, patients are started on empirical treatment with four first-line anti-TB drugs for the first 2 months of therapy. The patient then continues with two drugs, rifampicin and isoniazid, that are the two most effective anti-TB drugs currently available. Resistance to both rifampicin and isoniazid constitutes multidrug-resistant TB (MDR-TB). TB patients are monitored by microscopy and culture analysis of sputum. The first-line drugs usually initiated are rifampicin, isoniazid, pyrazinamide, and ethambutol, and the duration of standard treatment with these anti-TB drugs is 6 months. The duration of treatment may be prolonged in cases of extrapulmonary TB such as meningitis or spondylodiscitis. If drug-resistant TB is confirmed, or there is evidence that the patient acquired the disease from someone with confirmed resistant TB, such patients are treated with second-line anti-TB drugs [8].

Table 4.1 WHO classification of anti-TB drugs for longer multidrug-resistant tuberculosis (MDR-TB) regimens (communicated in August 2018)

Group	Agent	Comment
A	Levofloxacin or Moxifloxacin Bedaquiline Linezolid	Include all three medications except where contraindicated
B	Clofazimine Cycloserine or Terizidone	Add both medicines unless they cannot be used
C	Ethambutol Delamanid Pyrazinamide Imipenem–Cilastatin or Meropenem Amikacin or (streptomycin) Ethionamide/Protionamide p-Aminosalicylic acid	Add to complete regimen when drug in group A and B cannot be used

4.9 Drug Resistant-TB

Second-line TB drugs are much more expensive, they are given for longer periods, and have more severe side effects compared to first-line drugs. The WHO has been reviewing the treatment of drug-resistant TB based on resistant patterns from multiple centers. In August 2018, the WHO released a short communication on the treatment of rifampicin-resistant and multidrug-resistant TB [9]. Their recommendation for long-term use of TB drugs is summarized in Table 4.1 below. Previous WHO recommendations for shorter regimens of MDR-TB treatment classified anti-TB drugs into four groups: the fluoroquinolones, injectables, oral bacteriostatics, and add-ons, which appeared to be effective. Treatment for multidrug-resistant TB (MDR-TB) and extensively drug-resistant TB (XDR-TB) is becoming more individualized. XDR-TB is resistance to rifampicin, isoniazid, as well as at least one group A drug and one group B drug. The treatment options for XDR-TB are more challenging compared to the treatment of MDR-TB, with less success of treatment and increased mortality. In future, novel imaging possibilities with PET/CT may allow for the early identification of treatment resistance with appropriate early changes in management.

4.10 Surgery

Surgery was used in the treatment of TB before the advent of effective drugs. The role of surgery declined after TB drugs were discovered. In 2016, the WHO recommended the use of surgery in resistant TB and only in cases where the pulmonary disease is localized [10].

4.11   Side Effects

All TB medications have side effects that may be severe enough to result in the discontinuation of therapy. Most first-line TB drugs have hepatotoxicity as a known side effect, where monitoring the liver enzymes at baseline and during therapy is recommended. Isoniazid is associated with neuropathy (peripheral and central) and may result in seizures. The use of pyridoxine with isoniazid may reduce these effects and is also recommended for isoniazid-induced seizures. Linezolid may cause several side effects including anemia, bone marrow suppression, peripheral neuropathy, and lactic acidosis [11].

4.12   Drug Interactions

Some TB drugs may interact with other medications such as antiretroviral medication and may affect their efficacy, necessitating changes to either the antiretroviral or TB regimen. Rifampicin is a potent inducer of cytochrome P450 and is usually replaced by rifabutin in TB/HIV patients, as it is a less potent inducer of the liver enzymes.

4.13   Other Drugs Apart from Anti-TB

Certain types of TB such as TB meningitis may also benefit from the use of steroids. Pyridoxine is used to treat and prevent neuropathic side effects of some anti-TB medication.

4.14   Management of TB in HIV

The HIV disease has caused a resurgence of TB, especially in sub-Saharan Africa where TB is fueling the HIV pandemic. In the individual patient, TB drives the HIV to progress in the infection stage, causing HIV patients with TB to often present with atypical symptoms, more extrapulmonary involvement, or disseminated disease. It is important also to treat the HIV treat patients with TB/HIV coinfection. Multiple drug interactions may occur, and these may decrease their potency of some drugs. The increased pill burden may lead to a decrease in patient compliance that can potentially lead to resistant disease in either TB or HIV. HIV-immune reconstitution syndrome may unmask previously undiagnosed TB that may give rise to severe or even fatal TB, especially in patients with severe immunosuppression. Starting the antiretrovirals as soon as possible in TB/HIV coinfected patients improves the outcome. In patients who are severely immunosuppressed, it may be reasonable to start treatment of TB first at least for 8 weeks before the antiretroviral is started to prevent or reduce the effect of immune reconstitution [12].

4.15   Challenges in the Management of TB

Evidence-based treatment of susceptible TB is the best means of preventing drug resistance. TB treatment is prolonged, and patients may not adhere to the treatment resulting in recurrence and a possibility of development of drug resistance. Addition of a single agent to a failing regimen may also lead to drug resistance. Drug interaction with other conditions like HIV may lead to side effects or decrease the potency of other drugs [13]. Poor-quality TB drugs may also impact on the management of TB. To address some of these challenges the Directly Observed Treatment, Short-Course (DOTS) strategy was introduced. DOTS strategy includes direct government commitment, uninterrupted supply of essential TB drugs, and the direct supervision of taking the anti-TB drugs by the patient [14]. The DOTS strategy has also led to an increase in patient adherence. Extrapulmonary TB also presents unique challenges which may be addressed by PET/CT imaging options.

4.16   Conclusion

The management of TB should be a comprehensive one, which includes preventive measures and management of active TB. Prevention with vaccination in children is quite effective in contrast to the prevention of TB progression from latent infection in adults. Identification of such individuals with a high risk of progressing to active disease may in future be possible with novel PET imaging possibilities. Drug resistance and HIV can cause serious challenges to the management of infection and may lead to atypical-, extra-pulmonary, and more extensive involvement. Such individuals in particular may benefit from the ability of imaging with PET/CT to determine the extent of involvement, detect areas for biopsy, and to monitor treatment response.

References

1. World Health Organization. Global tuberculosis report 2018. Geneva: World Health Organization; 2018. p. 1–266.
2. Glaziou P, Floyd K, Raviglione MC. Global epidemiology of tuberculosis. Semin Respir Crit Care Med. 2018;39:271–85.
3. CDC. Treatment regimens for latent TB infection (LTBI). https://www.cdc.gov/tb/topic/treatment/ltbi.htm. Assessed on the 20th November 2018.
4. European Centre for Disease Control and Prevention. Tuberculosis prevention and control. https://ecdc.europa.eu/en/tuberculosis/prevention-and-control assessed on November 22, 2018.
5. WHO. Latent TB infection: updated and consolidated guidelines for programmatic management. Updated 2018. https://ecdc.europa.eu/en/tuberculosis/prevention-and-control assessed on November 25, 2018.

6. WHO policy on TB control in health-care facilities, congregate settings and households. World Health Organization 2009. p. 1–42.
7. Guidelines for the prevention of TB in health care facilities resource-limited settings. 1999 World Health Organization. pp 1–52.
8. Medscape. Herchline TE. Tuberculosis (TB) Treatment and Management. Updated October 31 2018 https://emedicine.medscape.com/article/230802-treatment assessed on November 20, 2018.
9. WHO. Key changes to the treatment of rifampicin-resistant and multi-drug resistant tuberculosis assessed December 15, 2018.
10. WHO treatment guidelines for drug resistant tuberculosis. 2016 update World Health Organization. p. 1–53.
11. Agyeman AA, Ofori-Asenso R. Efficacy and safety profile of linezolid in the treatment of multi-drug- resistant (MDR) and extensively drug-resistant (XDR) tuberculosis: a systemic review and meta-analysis. Ann Clin Microbiol Antimicrob. 2016;15:41.
12. Pawlowski A, Jansson M, Sköld M, Rottenberg ME, Källenius G. Tuberculosis HIV co-infection. PLoS Pathog. 2012;8(2):e1002464.
13. Egelund EF, Dupree L, Huesgen E, Peloquin CA. The pharmacological challenges of treating tuberculosis and HIV co-infection. Expert Rev Clin Pharmacol. 2017;10:213–23.
14. WHO. What is DOTS (Directly Observed Treatment, Short Course) http://www.searo.who.int/tb/topics/what_dots/en/ assessed December 3 2018.

FDG–PET Imaging in TB: Patient Preparation and Imaging

5

Vera Artiko and Jelena Pantovic

Contents

Fluorine-18-fluorodeoxyglucose (^{18}F-FDG)–positron emission tomography with computed tomography (PET/CT) is diagnostic tomographic imaging for the detection of metabolic activity in the human body. FDG is an analog of glucose which enters into viable cells via cell membrane glucose transporters (GLUT), especially GLUT1 and GLUT3, and phosphorylate with hexokinase inside cells. FDG is labeled with ^{18}F, which is a cyclotron-produced radioisotope with a half-life of 109.7 min that undergoes positron decay. The enhanced glucose consumption and subsequent higher ^{18}F-FDG uptake can be the result of high mitotic rates in malignances [1–3], granulomatous inflammation, and infection (sarcoidosis, fever of

V. Artiko (✉)
Faculty of Medicine, University of Belgrade, Belgrade, Serbia

Center for Nuclear Medicine, Clinical Center of Serbia, Belgrade, Serbia

J. Pantovic
Center for Nuclear Medicine, Clinical Center of Serbia, Belgrade, Serbia

© Springer Nature Switzerland AG 2020
D. Sobic Saranovic et al. (eds.), *PET/CT in Tuberculosis*, Clinicians' Guides to
Radionuclide Hybrid Imaging, https://doi.org/10.1007/978-3-030-47009-8_5

unknown origin, arthritis, tuberculosis and other infections, etc.) [4–6], tissue repair processes, a stress reaction of the affected cells in response to cell damage (metabolic flare) [7].

The ability of ^{18}F-FDG PET/CT to detect sites of inflammation and infection is based on the high glycolytic activity of the cells involved in the inflammatory response, especially neutrophils and the monocyte/macrophage family. Those cells in the active sites of inflammation/infection express high levels of GLUT1 and GLUT3 as well as hexokinase activity [8, 9]. Based on high level of metabolism and glycolytic activity in granulomatous inflammation, active tuberculosis (TB) sites induce an accumulation of ^{18}F-FDG [10, 11] and subsequently can be detected by PET/CT.

Standardization of PET/CT procedure is important to enable use of metabolic parameters as imaging biomarkers in routine clinical practice, ensure reproducibility, and allow comparative examinations across different nuclear medicine sites.

Nuclear medicine physician's justification of the clinical request for ^{18}F-FDG PET/CT in patients with TB is important (for assessment of activity in tuberculosis lesions, detection of extrapulmonary sites of infection, and evaluation of therapy response) [12] because of lower level of evidence (Cochrane C and D) for these indications.

5.1 Patient Preparation

The aim of patient preparation for ^{18}F-FDG PET/CT is to minimize dietary glucose-related competitive inhibition of ^{18}F-FDG uptake in the viable cells and reduce serum insulin level to near basal level. In addition, it is important to minimize tracer uptake in normal tissue (myocardium, skeletal muscles, and urinary track) and maintain uptake in target tissue [13].

5.1.1 One or Two Days Before Scanning

Therefore, low-carbohydrate high-protein diet, physical activity restriction [14] (strenuous exercise and housework), as well as the restriction of deep tissue massage are recommended 24–48 h before scanning.

5.1.2 On the Day of Scanning

Patient should be instructed to fast for at least 4–6 h before the administration of ^{18}F-FDG, to decrease physiologic glucose levels and to reduce serum insulin level to near basal levels. Oral hydration with water is encouraged to ensure hydration and promote diuresis.

Necessary medications are allowed and must be recorded. Some medication could interfere with quality of PET scan: elevating glucose plasma level (steroids, glucocorticoids, lithium, ephedrine, etc.) or increasing the accumulation of ^{18}F-FDG in bowel (metformin) [15, 16] (Fig. 5.1).

In diabetic patients who received insulin early in the morning, the scan may be scheduled 3–4 h after breakfast.

5.2 Clinical Evaluation by the Nuclear Medicine Physician Before ^{18}F-FDG Injection

The nuclear medicine physician should have available all information that could facilitate the interpretation of ^{18}F-FDG imaging (CT, magnetic resonance imaging—MRI, and other previously performed diagnostic imaging, including any previous PET/CT study). It is important to check fasting state of the patients, diabetic history, record the prescribed mediation and presence of fever or elevation of acute inflammatory markers, recent trauma, surgery or invasive diagnostic procedure, and history of malignant or benign disease with high tissue proliferation. Suspected or confirmed pregnancy is contraindicated for examination; there is no recommendation for interruption of breastfeeding after administration of ^{18}F-FDG since it excretes little through milk [17]. However, the recommendation is that contact between mother and child should be limited for 12 h after injection of ^{18}F-FDG to reduce the radiation dose that the infant receives from external exposure from the mother.

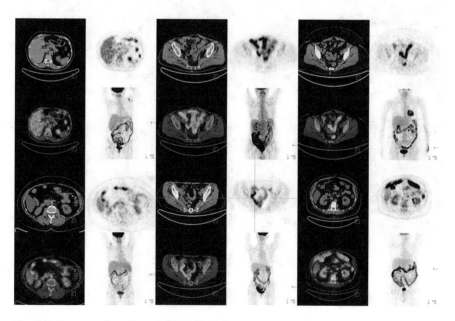

Fig. 5.1 Few examples of bowel ^{18}F-FDG uptake in patients with metformin therapy

5.3   Prior to the Injection of ¹⁸F-FDG

Patient weight and height should be check for two reasons: to calculate weight-based dose for radiopharmaceutical administration and for semiquantitative assessment of ¹⁸F-FDG uptake in the lesions.

Glucose plasma level should be measured and physiological or less than 10 mmol/l is desirable to prevent glucose-related competitive inhibition of ¹⁸F-FDG uptake in the target tissue.

Relaxation and warm room environment half an hour or an hour before tracer injection will prevent and/or reduce ¹⁸F-FDG brown fat uptake especially in young patients. In some patients, additional relaxation is necessary using oral dose of diazepam or beta-blockers to reduce undesirable uptake in brown fat and muscles [18, 19] (Fig. 5.2).

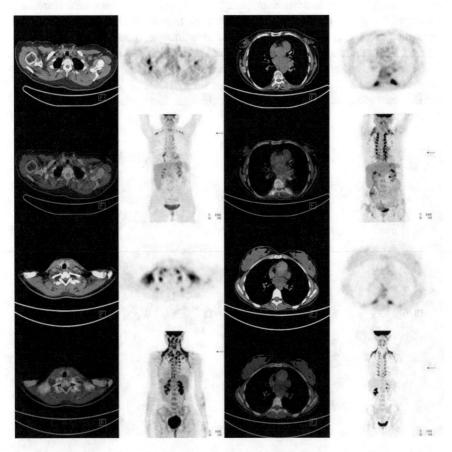

Fig. 5.2 Two examples of ¹⁸F-FDG uptake in brown fat in adults (first row) and in young patients (second row)

It is also important to remove all metal (jewelry, dental braces, clothes with metal zippers) that could lead to streak artifacts on CT transmission scan.

5.4 Intravenous Injection of ^{18}F-FDG and Uptake Period After Injection

According to the European Association of Nuclear Medicine–Society of Nuclear Medicine and Molecular Imaging (EANM SNMMI) Guidelines [13], calculated dose for imaging depends on the body weight and age of the patient, as well as on the sensitivity of hybrid PET/CT scanner and is most commonly in the range of 2.5–5.5 MBq/kg of ^{18}F-FDG. After administration of radiopharmaceutical, the patient should stay relaxed (seated or laying) to avoid muscular uptake. Patients are encouraged to drink 1l of still water while waiting for scanning and advise to empty bladder immediately before the acquisition to limit the radiation dose to the renal collecting system and clear pelvis region on the PET scan.

Acquisition usually starts 60 min after intravenous (iv) injection of ^{18}F-FDG. This interval allows adequate time for intracellular uptake, trapping of the radiopharmaceutical, and its clearance from the blood.

5.5 Image Acquisition

Patients are positioned comfortably on the examination table (pallet) with their arms raised above the head if that position can be tolerated by the patient, and should be supported with adequate positioning aids (knee, head and neck, arm support) to limit involuntary motion that may lead to general or local misalignment during the combined examination. Arms along the side may produce beam-hardening artifacts over the torso. The acquisition is usually performed as whole body mode from the base of the skull, or top of the skull, to the proximal thighs (Fig. 5.3).

It starts with a CT topogram. The topogram is used to define the axial examination range of the PET/CT study. CT acquisition begins after the definition of the coaxial imaging range, and the patient is moved automatically into the CT field of view for the transmission scan. Most PET/CT users acquire a single continuous spiral CT scan. After the completion of the CT scan, the patient is advanced to the field of view of the PET using a step of 1.5–3 min per bed position starting from pelvic area when the bladder is empty (Fig. 5.4).

Typically, for skull to mid-thigh imaging, the total acquisition time ranges from 15 to 40 min. The imaging time is typically prolonged for the acquisition of brain images or for images of a limited region of interest.

Some centers recommend *dual-time-point acquisition* with early (60 min after iv injection of ^{18}F-FDG) and late scanning (90–120 min after iv injection of ^{18}F-FDG) to better differentiate between active TB and malignant lesions [20, 21]. Malignant

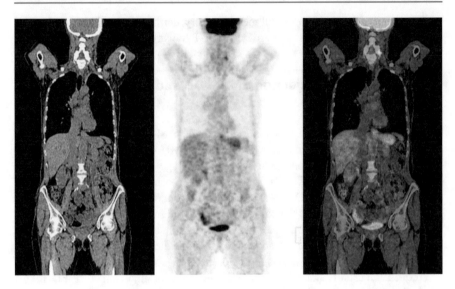

Fig. 5.3 Optimal patient position (arms raised above the head) during PET and CT imaging

Fig. 5.4 Bed positions on topogram (arms raised above the head) that are used to define the axial examination range of the PET/CT study

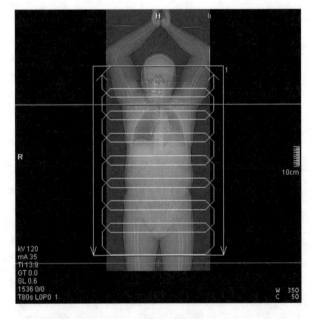

tissue may continue to concentrate on the tracer with the time and the background will continue to decrease. By contrast active TB lesions may show "wash out" activity with time (Fig. 5.5). However, from the literature, dual-time acquisition does not reliably help in the distinguishing active TB from malignant tumor tissue [20].

Fig. 5.5 ¹⁸F-FDG accumulation in malignant and inflammatory cells. Malignant tissue shows increasing levels of ¹⁸F-FDG uptake in a function of time, while peak of ¹⁸F-FDG accumulation in inflammatory tissue is around 60 min after the injection and then decreases gradually

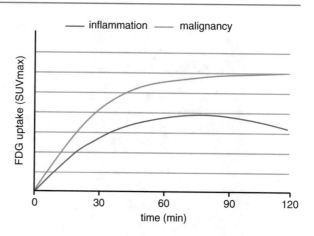

5.6   Image Analysis and Interpretation

Post-acquisition reconstruction sets contain CT data as well as corrected and non-corrected PET data.

In addition, several post-acquisition reconstruction tasks may be required to create CT image sets with alternate filter and window levels (e.g., lung, bone, parenchyma windows).

Special viewing and fusion tools typically are available with standard PET/CT software to allow through any of the selected individual and fused image volumes as well as side-by-side viewing. The software packages usually provide registered and aligned CT images, PET images, and fusion images (in the axial, coronal, and sagittal planes), as well as maximum-intensity projection (MIP) images for review in the 3D mode (Fig. 5.6). ¹⁸F-FDG PET images with and without attenuation correction should be available for review.

In the imaging analysis and interpretation it is important to be aware of physiological distribution of ¹⁸F-FDG that is seen in the brain, heart, kidney and urinary system, and thymus (in children and young patients) on the PET scan. Physiological activity can vary in the lymphoid tissue of the Waldeyer ring and in gastrointestinal system, especially in bowel [22, 23].

Visual, qualitative analysis means looking for increased, not physiological, ¹⁸F-FDG uptake in whole body PET scan. It is important to take into account pattern of uptake (focal, diffuse, linear, etc.) and intensity, and morphological information obtain by CT.

Quantitative parameters, such as standardized uptake values (*SUVmax*), are calculated using the following formula:

$$SUVmax = tissue\ concentration\,(MBq\,/\,g)\,/\,\big[\,injected\ dose\,(MBq)\,/\,body\ weight\,\big].$$

SUVmax should be used with caution in patients with TB because it is not yet validated in literature and clinical practice. However, it could be of value for monitoring the response of the disease to the therapy [24, 25].

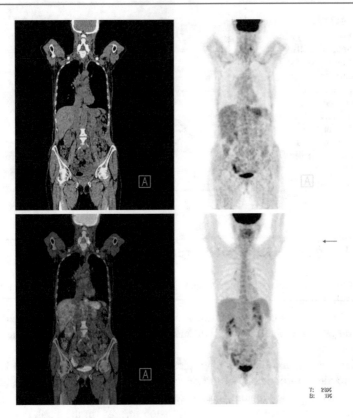

Fig. 5.6 CT, PET, fusion image (PET/CT), and MIP

References

1. Artiko V, Odalovic S, Sobic-Saranovic D, Petrovic M, Stojiljkovic M, Petrovic N, Kozarevic N, Grozdic-Milojevic I, Obradovic V. Can (18)F-FDG PET/CT scan change treatment planning and be prognostic in recurrent colorectal carcinoma? A prospective and follow-up study. Hell J Nucl Med. 2015;18(1):35–41.
2. Boellaard R, O'Doherty MJ, Weber WA, et al. FDG PET and PET/CT: EANM procedure guidelines for tumor PET imaging: version 1.0. Eur J Nucl Med Mol Imaging. 2010;37:181–200.
3. Sobic Saranovic D, Stojiljkovic M, Susnjar S, Odalovic S, Artiko V, Pavlovic S, Grozdic-Milojevic I. Obradovic metabolic activity of breast cancer metastatic lesions on positron emission tomography/computed tomography: comparison with histological and biological characteristics of primary tumor. Neoplasma. 2016;63(2):313–21.
4. Mortimer JE, Dehdashti F, Siegal BA, et al. Metabolic flare: indicator of hormone responsiveness in advanced breast cancer. J Clin Oncol. 2001;19:2797–803.
5. Saponjski J, Sobic-Saranovic D, Odalovic S, Stojiljković M, Pantovic J, Petrovic N, Grozdic-Milojevic I, Artiko V. The detection of endocarditis, post implantation grafts, arteritis and other related disorders by ^{18}F-FDG PET/CT. Hell J Nucl Med. 2017;20(Suppl):37–44.
6. Sobic-Saranovic D, Artiko V, Obradovic V. FDG PET imaging in sarcoidosis. Semin Nucl Med. 2013;43:404–11.

7. Mochizuki T, Tsukamoto E, Kuge Y, et al. FDG uptake and glucose transporter subtype expressions in experimental tumor and inflammation models. J Nucl Med. 2001;42:1551–5.
8. Gamelli RL, Liu H, He LK, Hofmann CA. Augmentations of glucose uptake and glucose transporter-1 in macrophages following thermal injury and sepsis in mice. J Leukoc Biol. 1996;59:639–47.
9. Vorster M, Sathekge MM, Bomanji J. Advances in imaging of tuberculosis: the role of ^{18}F-FDG PET and PET/CT. Curr Opin Pulm Med. 2014;20:287–93.
10. Ankrah AO, Glaudemans AWJM, Maes A, Van de Wiele C, Dierckx RAJO, Vorster M, Sathekge MM. Tuberculosis. Semin Nucl Med. 2018;48:108–30.
11. Martinez V, Castilla-Lievre MA, Guillet-Caruba C, Grenier G, Fior R, Desarnaud S, Doucet-Populaire F, Boué F. (18)F-FDG PET/CT in tuberculosis: an early non-invasive marker of therapeutic response. Int J Tuberc Lung Dis. 2012;16:1180–5.
12. Surasi DS, Bhambhvani P, Baldwin JA, Almodovar SE, O'Malley JP. 18F-FDG PET and PET/CT patient preparation: a review of the literature. J Nucl Med Technol. 2014;42:5–13.
13. Jamar F, Buscombe J, Chiti A, Christian PE, Delbeke D, Donohoe KJ, Israel O, Comin JM, Signore A. EANM/SNMMI guideline for 18F-FDG use in inflammation and infection. J Nucl Med. 2013;54:647–58.
14. Oh JR, Song HC, Chong A, et al. Impact of medication discontinuation on increased intestinal FDG accumulation in diabetic patients treated with metformin. AJR. 2010;195:1404–10.
15. Gontier E, Fourme E, Wartski M, et al. High and typical ^{18}F-FDG bowel uptake in patients treated with metformin. Eur J Nucl Med Mol Imaging. 2008;35:95–9.
16. ICRP. Radiation dose to patients from radiopharmaceuticals: addendum 3 to ICRP publication 53—ICRP publication 106. Approved by the Commission in October 2007. Ann ICRP. 2008;38:1–197.
17. Cohade C. Altered biodistribution of FDG-PET with emphasis on brown fat and insulin effect. Semin Nucl Med. 2010;40:283–93.
18. Agrawal A, Nair N, Baghel NS. A novel approach for reduction of brown fat uptake on FDG PET. Br J Radiol. 2009;82:626–31.
19. Lan XL, Zhang YX, Wu ZJ, et al. The value of dual time point (18)F-FDG PET imaging for the differentiation between malignant and benign lesions. Clin Radiol. 2008;63(7):756–64.
20. Houshmand S, Salavati A, Segtnan EA, Grupe P, Høilund-Carlsen PF, Alavi A. Dual-time-point imaging and delayed-time-point Fluorodeoxyglucose-PET/computed tomography imaging in various clinical setting. PET Clin. 2016;11:65–84.
21. Schillaci O. Use of dual-point fluorodeoxyglucose imaging to enhance sensitivity and specificity. Semin Nucl Med. 2012;42:267–80.
22. Cook GJ, Fogelman I, Maisey MN. Normal physiology and benign pathological variants of 18-fluoro-2-deoxyglucose positron emission tomography scanning: potential for error in interpretation. Semin Nucl Med. 1996;26:308–14.
23. Shammas A, Lim R, Charron M. Pediatric FDG PET/CT: physiologic uptake, normal variants, and benign conditions. Radiographics. 2009;29:1467–86.
24. Gambhir S, Ravina M, Rangan K, Dixit M, Barai S, Bomanji J, the International Atomic Energy Agency Extra-pulmonary TB Consortium (Sobic Saranovic D). Imaging in extrapulmonary tuberculosis. Int J Infect Dis. 2017;56:237–47.
25. Martin C, Castaigne C, Vierasu I, Garcia C, Wyndham-Thomas C, de Wit S. Prospective serial FDG PET/CT during treatment of Extrapulmonary tuberculosis in HIV-infected patients: an exploratory study. Clin Nucl Med. 2018;43:635–40.

FDG PET in Pulmonary TB: Current Evidence

6

T. Lengana and Mariza Vorster

Contents

6.1   Introduction

Positron emission tomography (PET) with ^{18}F-fluorodeoxyglucose (^{18}F-FDG) has evolved from its established role in oncology to also have an impact in infection imaging. Cells involved in infection and inflammation (mainly neutrophils and monocytes) demonstrate increased ^{18}F-FDG accumulation due a combination of factors, which include increased expression of Glucose Transporter (GLUT) transporters and hexokinase as well as increased aerobic oxidation [1]. The imaging of these metabolic changes in infection is superior to anatomical imaging in that metabolic changes will commence prior to the structural changes in response to infection, and will also resolve earlier. This provides the potential for early detection of infection and accurate assessment of treatment response with metabolic imaging

T. Lengana (✉) · M. Vorster
Department of Nuclear Medicine, University of Pretoria & Steve Biko Academic Hospital, Pretoria, South Africa

© Springer Nature Switzerland AG 2020
D. Sobic Saranovic et al. (eds.), *PET/CT in Tuberculosis*, Clinicians' Guides to Radionuclide Hybrid Imaging, https://doi.org/10.1007/978-3-030-47009-8_6

[2]. Some of the infection imaging applications of ^{18}F-FDG include its use in fever of unknown origin, sarcoidosis, vasculitis, bone infections, vascular graft infection, diabetic foot infection, assessment of treatment response in infective and inflammatory conditions, TB and HIV applications [1, 3, 4].

With regards to pulmonary TB, the use of FDG PET/CT imaging has been investigated in the following settings: characterizing pulmonary nodules, distinguishing of tuberculous lesions from malignant ones (making use of various SUV_{max} cut-off values and Dual Time Point Imaging), distinguishing latent from active TB, and in treatment response evaluation.

The granuloma forms a central part of the pathophysiology of tuberculosis and consists of various immune cells that are initially representative of innate immunity and which at a later stage stimulate the processes involved in adaptive immunity. TB granulomas are dynamic structures with lymphocyte movements that are similar to those found with lymph nodes. The early granulomas promote phagocytosis of infected macrophages and secrete matrix metallopeptidase 9 (MMP-9), which in turn stimulates chemotaxis of new macrophages. As such, it provides multiple targets for imaging.

6.2 Pulmonary TB and FDG Uptake Patterns

Pulmonary TB has been classified into two types, primary and post-primary (reactivation), which are based on typical radiological findings [5]. Primary TB is seen at initial exposure to the *mycobacterium bacillus* and may demonstrate multi-lobar consolidation that may either resolve or evolve to a radiological scar or opacity (tuberculoma). Post-primary TB will typically demonstrate consolidation in the upper lobes or superior segments of the lower lobes with associated cavitation [6].

Two patterns of ^{18}F-FDG uptake have been described in the imaging of pulmonary TB—the lung and the lymphatic pattern of uptake. The lung pattern consists of limited, mildly metabolically active areas of lung consolidation and/or cavities and is mainly seen in patients with pulmonary symptoms (See Figs. 6.1–6.3). The lymphatic pattern, on the other hand, comprises of significantly increased extrapulmonary metabolically active lesions, including mediastinal lymph nodes and extrathoracic lymph nodes, and these patients mainly present with systemic symptoms [7] (see Fig. 6.4).

The aforementioned patterns of uptake are mainly a result of the host immune status. Patients who are immune competent are more likely to demonstrate the lung pattern, while those who are immune incompetent are more likely to present with the lymphatic pattern [8, 9].

Pulmonary tuberculomas will typically demonstrate increased metabolic activity on ^{18}F-FDG PET. Goo et al. reviewed imaging with ^{18}F-FDG in a series of 10 patients with pulmonary tuberculomas. The researchers were able to demonstrate increased metabolic activity in 9 out of the 10 granulomas, with a mean SUV_{max} value of 4.2 (range 1.9–3.7) [10].

Fig. 6.1 ^{18}F-FDG PET/CT image demonstrating intense uptake in active pulmonary TB with cavitations and consolidation noted on CT

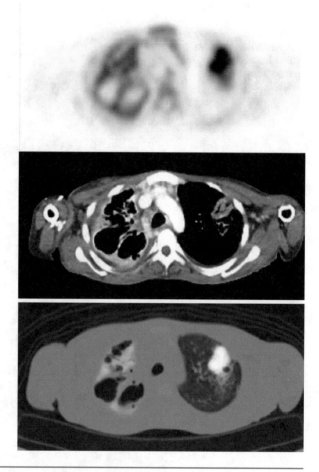

6.3   Comparisons Between ^{18}F-FDG PET and Computed Tomography (CT)

In a series by Sathekge et al., reviewing the impact of ^{18}F-FDG PET on the management of tuberculosis treatment, 16 patients with active tuberculosis were included. Patients underwent contrast-enhanced computed tomography (CT) and ^{18}F-FDG PET at 45 and 120 min. Early and delayed SUV_{max} values and the percentage change in SUV values were obtained. CT and ^{18}F-FDG PET identified the same number of lesions in the lungs, with a mean early image SUV_{max} of 8.2 (range 3.4–21.7). ^{18}F-FDG however identified double the number of lymph nodes when compared to CT, with a mean SUV_{max} of 6.3 (range 3.4–9.2). Other sites of involvement included pleural, osseous, and joint involvement and interestingly ^{18}F-FDG detected additional sites missed by CT, which had an impact on treatment duration [11].

In a study by Stelzmueller et al., 35 patients were included in an assessment of the value of ^{18}F-FDG in the initial evaluation of patients with tuberculosis. Features

Fig. 6.2 A 45-year-old
female with newly
diagnosed TB. ^{18}F-FDG
PET image demonstrates
diffuse bilateral
metabolically active TB
involvement

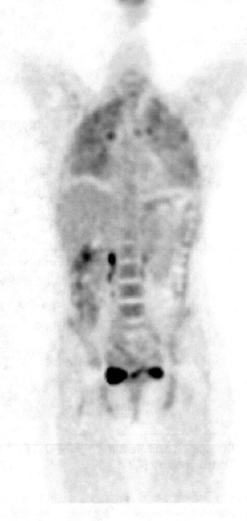

of infection on ^{18}F-FDG PET were compared to those on CT. PET imaging was able
to detect 64 affected areas in 23 patients, while CT only detected 34 affected areas,
highlighting ^{18}F-FDG PET's role in accurately assessing disease extent [12].

Similarly 47 patients with pulmonary mycobacteriosis underwent high-resolution
CT and ^{18}F-FDG PET studies to assess pulmonary disease activity and to determine
treatment response. Lesion SUV_{max} and visual assessments were compared to high-
resolution CT findings. Of these patients 22 had tuberculosis while 25 had mycobacterium avium-intracellulare complex. Using a cut-off SUV_{max} of 4.0, ^{18}F-FDG
demonstrated an accuracy of 100% in distinguishing active from inactive pulmonary mycobacteriosis in a comparison with high-resolution CT images (which were

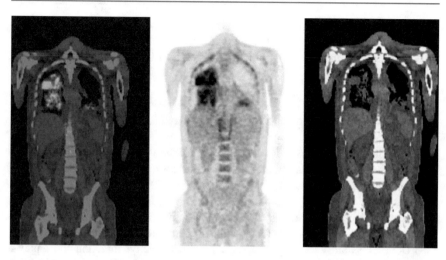

Fig. 6.3 ^{18}F-FDG PET/CT images demonstrating bilateral metabolically active consolidation in a 28-year-old patient with newly diagnosed TB

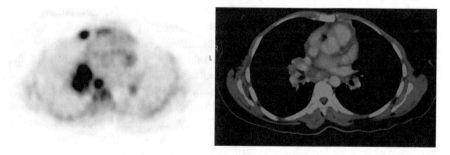

Fig. 6.4 ^{18}F-FDG PET/CT image demonstrating intense uptake in mediastinal lymph nodes in an immune-compromised patient

positive for active disease). Lesions which did not demonstrate active TB on high-resolution CT demonstrated a reduced metabolic activity on PET. ^{18}F-FDG PET, however, was not able to reliably distinguish between active tuberculosis and active mycobacterium avium-intracellulare complex lesions [13].

6.4 Dual Time Point Imaging

Kim et al. investigated the usefulness of ^{18}F-FDG dual time point imaging in distinguishing active from inactive pulmonary tuberculosis lesions. Twenty-five patients with tuberculoma were included in the study and were imaged at 60 and 120 min post tracer injection. Lesion activity was determined based on a visual score, early and delayed SUV_{max} values, and the percentage change of SUV_{max} from early to delayed. They found that active tuberculosis could be differentiated from inactive tuberculosis with 100% sensitivity and 100% specificity when using an early SUV_{max} cut-off value of 1.05, while the delayed SUV_{max} cut-off value of 0.97 yielded a sensitivity of 92.8%, and specificity of 100% [14].

6.5   Distinguishing Between Active and Latent TB

Not all patients with exposure to *Mycobacterium tuberculosis* will develop symptomatic TB with the typical night sweats, weight loss, and fever. More often than not, immune-competent patients will develop latent TB, where active TB infection is prevented by the patients' immune system [15, 16]. In the management of TB, it is imperative that patients at risk of developing active tuberculosis are identified so that preventative measures may be taken, and treatment can be initiated early [17]. ^{18}F-FDG PET's ability to image molecular changes in active infection could play a vital role in identifying these patients who could be at risk for progressing from latent tuberculosis to active infection.

Lin et al. studied 26 cynomolgus macaques with latent tuberculosis. ^{18}F-FDG PET imaging of the macaque prior to the administration of TNF-neutralizing antibody was able to predict reactivation with 92% sensitivity and specificity. Some of the ^{18}F-FDG PET features which have been identified as risk factors for the development of active infection include increased total lung ^{18}F-FDG avidity, granuloma $SUV_{max} \geq 5$, and the presence of extra-pulmonary lesions [18].

Ghesani et al. conducted a study to determine if ^{18}F-FDG PET could detect early events in latent TB. Five patients who had been in close proximity to pulmonary TB-positive patients were included. Latent TB was confirmed by the following: no signs or symptoms of active TB, no radiological features of active TB, and positive QuantiFERON gold assay. Baseline ^{18}F-FDG PET/CT imaging was done on four of the five patients. The positive scans demonstrated metabolically active thoracic nodal uptake which were not radiologically significant without any lung parenchymal uptake [19].

6.6   Distinguishing Benign from Malignant Lung Lesions

It is well known that malignant cells demonstrate increased glucose utilization, which can be imaged with ^{18}F-FDG. This poses an imaging dilemma in infection imaging as ^{18}F-FDG may be unable to differentiate infection or inflammation from malignancy [20]. The pulmonary tuberculoma is one of the more common pulmonary nodules and contributes significantly to the benign pulmonary nodules which are excised to exclude malignancy [21].

Dual time point imaging has also been used in this setting as a means to differentiate infection from malignancy. It is anticipated that malignant cells will continue to concentrate ^{18}F-FDG over time while infective/inflammatory cells will initially peak and then slowly start to reduce ^{18}F-FDG concentration [22, 23].

Chen et al. reviewed the usefulness of ^{18}F-FDG dual time point imaging in a total of 31 lesions with an initial SUV_{max} <2.5, assessing whether delayed imaging would improve the accuracy in differentiating benign from malignant primary nodules. They found that both benign and malignant pulmonary lesions demonstrated an increase in SUV_{max} and retention indexes of >10%. Sensitivity and specificity for ^{18}F-FDG PET was 62% and 40% respectively when a retention index of >10% for malignancy was used and there was no statistical difference between the retention indexes of the benign versus malignant pulmonary nodules ($p = 0.8$) [24].

In the assessment of solitary pulmonary nodules in 30 patients from a tuberculosis endemic environment, Sathekge et al. found that ^{18}F-FDG dual time point imaging was not able to differentiate between malignant nodules versus those due to tuberculoma. Using an SUV_{max} cut off of 2.5, ^{18}F-FDG PET only yielded a sensitivity and specificity of 85.7% and 25% respectively while using a change in SUV_{max} of >10% yielded a sensitivity and specificity of 85.7% and 50% respectively. ^{18}F-FDG PET specificity for SUV_{max} cut off of 2.5 and percentage change of >10% as an indicator for malignancy only increased with the removal of the TB patients from the analyzed data to 100% and 75% respectively. Interestingly they found that the rate of increase of SUV_{max} did not differ significantly between malignant lesions and tuberculoma. They concluded that dual time point imaging could not reliably differentiate between benign and malignant lung lesions in regions where TB is endemic [25].

Similarly Kaneko et al. reviewed 81 lung lesions with an SUV_{max} >2.5 and diameter > 10 mm, of which 47 were due to primary lung cancer and the rest due to benign conditions, including tuberculoma. They compared the differences in FDG retention in the benign versus malignant lesions and in tuberculous versus non-tuberculous benign pulmonary lesions using dual time point imaging. They found that there was no statistically significant difference between the SUV change of the malignant versus those of the benign lesions ($p = 0.95$). Interestingly, this group also could not demonstrate a statistically significant difference in SUV change between the tuberculous lesions versus other non-tuberculous benign pulmonary lesions ($p = 0.93$). The researchers concluded that while the cellular mechanisms for the increasing ^{18}F-FDG retention in tuberculoma are not clearly understood, GLUT 1 expression may play a role [26].

6.7   In Summary

- Two patterns of ^{18}F-FDG uptake have been described in pulmonary tuberculosis, which is dependent on the host immune status. The lung pattern is associated with pulmonary symptoms in immune-competent patients and the more extensive lymphatic pattern, which is associated with systemic illness, is seen in immune-compromised individuals.
- The molecular metabolic findings that are inherent to PET imaging may be more useful in particular settings when compared to those of morphological imaging modalities as metabolic changes tend to precede morphological ones. This may

be particularly useful when evaluating treatment response and in distinguishing active TB from latent TB.

- Dual time point imaging depends on the well-described different washout rates between infective lesions and malignant ones. Although it has shown some promise in distinguishing active from inactive disease, this imaging technique has not convincingly demonstrated acceptable accuracy in distinguishing benign from malignant lesions and is certainly not recommended in areas where TB is endemic.
- It would be clinically useful to be able to predict which patients are likely to progress from latent to active TB. Total lung ^{18}F-FDG avidity, granuloma SUV ≥ 5, and the presence of extrapulmonary lesions have all been identified as promising predictors in this setting.

References

1. Jamar F, Buscombe J, Chiti A, Christian PE, Delbeke D, Donohoe KJ, et al. EANM/SNMMI guideline for 18F-FDG use in inflammation and infection. J Nucl Med. 2013;54:647–58.
2. Lawal I, Zeevaart J, Ebenhan T, Ankrah A, Vorster M, Kruger HG, et al. Metabolic imaging of infection. J Nucl Med. 2017;58:1727–32.
3. Glaudemans AW, Signore A. FDG-PET/CT in infections: the imaging method of choice? Eur J Nucl Med Mol Imaging. 2010;37:1986–91.
4. Vaidyanathan S, Patel CN, Scarsbrook AF, Chowdhury FU. FDG PET/CT in infection and inflammation—current and emerging clinical applications. Clin Radiol. 2015;70:787–800.
5. Van Dyck P, Vanhoenacker FM, Van den Brande P, De Schepper AM. Imaging of pulmonary tuberculosis. Eur Radiol. 2003;13:1771–85.
6. Bomanji JB, Gupta N, Gulati P, Das CJ. Imaging in tuberculosis. Cold Spring Harb Perspect Med. 2015;5:a017814.
7. Soussan M, Brillet PY, Mekinian A, Khafagy A, Nicolas P, Vessieres A, et al. Patterns of pulmonary tuberculosis on FDG-PET/CT. Eur J Radiol. 2012;81:2872–6.
8. Rizzi EB, Schinina V, Palmieri F, Girardi E, Bibbolino C. Radiological patterns in HIV-associated pulmonary tuberculosis: comparison between HAART-treated and non-HAART-treated patients. Clin Radiol. 2003;58:469–73.
9. Geng E, Kreiswirth B, Burzynski J, Schluger NW. Clinical and radiographic correlates of primary and reactivation tuberculosis: a molecular epidemiology study. JAMA. 2005;293:2740–5.
10. Goo JM, Im JG, Do KH, Yeo JS, Seo JB, Kim HY, et al. Pulmonary tuberculoma evaluated by means of FDG PET: findings in 10 cases. Radiology. 2000;216:117–21.
11. Sathekge M, Maes A, Kgomo M, Stoltz A, Pottel H, Van de Wiele C. Impact of FDG PET on the management of TBC treatment. A pilot study. Nuklearmedizin. 2010;49:35–40.
12. Stelzmueller I, Huber H, Wunn R, Hodolic M, Mandl M, Lamprecht B, et al. 18F-FDG PET/CT in the initial assessment and for follow-up in patients with tuberculosis. Clin Nucl Med. 2016;41:e187–94.
13. Demura Y, Tsuchida T, Uesaka D, Umeda Y, Morikawa M, Ameshima S, et al. Usefulness of 18F-fluorodeoxyglucose positron emission tomography for diagnosing disease activity and monitoring therapeutic response in patients with pulmonary mycobacteriosis. Eur J Nucl Med Mol Imaging. 2009;36:632–9.
14. Kim IJ, Lee JS, Kim SJ, Kim YK, Jeong YJ, Jun S, et al. Double-phase 18F-FDG PET-CT for determination of pulmonary tuberculoma activity. Eur J Nucl Med Mol Imaging. 2008;35:808–14.

15. Salgame P, Geadas C, Collins L, Jones-Lopez E, Ellner JJ. Latent tuberculosis infection—revisiting and revising concepts. Tuberculosis (Edinb). 2015;95:373–84.
16. Dheda K, Barry CE 3rd, Maartens G. Tuberculosis. Lancet. 2016;387:1211–26.
17. Horsburgh CR Jr. Priorities for the treatment of latent tuberculosis infection in the United States. N Engl J Med. 2004;350:2060–7.
18. Lin PL, Maiello P, Gideon HP, Coleman MT, Cadena AM, Rodgers MA, et al. PET CT identifies reactivation risk in Cynomolgus macaques with latent M. tuberculosis. PLoS Pathog. 2016;12:e1005739.
19. Ghesani N, Patrawalla A, Lardizabal A, Salgame P, Fennelly KP. Increased cellular activity in thoracic lymph nodes in early human latent tuberculosis infection. Am J Respir Crit Care Med. 2014;189:748–50.
20. Mamede M, Higashi T, Kitaichi M, Ishizu K, Ishimori T, Nakamoto Y, et al. [18F]FDG uptake and PCNA, Glut-1, and hexokinase-II expressions in cancers and inflammatory lesions of the lung. Neoplasia. 2005;7:369–79.
21. Kikano GE, Fabien A, Schilz R. Evaluation of the solitary pulmonary nodule. Am Fam Physician. 2015;92:1084–91.
22. Zhuang H, Pourdehnad M, Lambright ES, Yamamoto AJ, Lanuti M, Li P, et al. Dual time point 18F-FDG PET imaging for differentiating malignant from inflammatory processes. J Nucl Med. 2001;42:1412–7.
23. Schillaci O. Use of dual-point fluorodeoxyglucose imaging to enhance sensitivity and specificity. Semin Nucl Med. 2012;42:267–80.
24. Chen CJ, Lee BF, Yao WJ, Cheng L, Wu PS, Chu CL, et al. Dual-phase 18F-FDG PET in the diagnosis of pulmonary nodules with an initial standard uptake value less than 2.5. AJR Am J Roentgenol. 2008;191:475–9.
25. Sathekge MM, Maes A, Pottel H, Stoltz A, van de Wiele C. Dual time-point FDG PET-CT for differentiating benign from malignant solitary pulmonary nodules in a TB endemic area. S Afr Med J. 2010;100:598–601.
26. Kaneko K, Sadashima E, Irie K, Hayashi A, Masunari S, Yoshida T, et al. Assessment of FDG retention differences between the FDG-avid benign pulmonary lesion and primary lung cancer using dual-time-point FDG-PET imaging. Ann Nucl Med. 2013;27:392–9.

FDG PET/CT in Extrapulmonary TB: Current Evidence

7

Dragana Sobic Saranovic, Jelena Saponjski, and Dragica Pesut

Contents

According to the World Health Organization, extrapulmonary tuberculosis is defined as bacteriologically, histologically, or clinically diagnosed tuberculosis that involves organs other than the lungs, such as pleura, lymph nodes, abdomen, genitourinary tract, skin, joints and bones, and meninges. Also considered to be extrapulmonary

D. Sobic Saranovic (✉)
Faculty of Medicine, University of Belgrade, Belgrade, Serbia

Center for Nuclear Medicine, Clinical Center of Serbia, Belgrade, Serbia

J. Saponjski
Center for Nuclear Medicine, Clinical Center of Serbia, Belgrade, Serbia

D. Pesut
Faculty of Medicine, University of Belgrade, Belgrade, Serbia

Clinic for Lung Diseases, Clinical Center of Serbia, Belgrade, Serbia

© Springer Nature Switzerland AG 2020
D. Sobic Saranovic et al. (eds.), *PET/CT in Tuberculosis*, Clinicians' Guides to Radionuclide Hybrid Imaging, https://doi.org/10.1007/978-3-030-47009-8_7

tuberculosis is a case of tuberculous lymphadenopathy (mediastinal, hilar) or tuberculous pleural effusion, without radiographic abnormalities in the lungs, unlike the cases with both pulmonary and extrapulmonary tuberculosis that are classified as pulmonary alone [1].

Extrapulmonary tuberculosis is more common in elderly patients, children, as well as in those with immunodeficiency (HIV; malignant diseases such as lymphoma, leukaemia, etc.; and those on immunosuppressive medication). Depending on which organ system is affected, tuberculosis varies in clinical symptomatology and radiological findings. Patients with extensive or a coexisting disease may experience systemic symptoms such as fever, night sweats, fatigue, and loss of appetite and body weight, so it can mimic numerous disease entities [2, 3]. Further diagnosis is made based on clinical history, positive microbiological cultures, histological confirmation, positive tuberculin test which supports the diagnosis (but negative does not exclude it), serological analyses, thorax X-rays, and CT. Histopathological verification after the specimen biopsy or tumor/lymph node extirpation is sometimes needed for definitive diagnosis [4–6].

^{18}F-FDG PET/CT plays an important role in the evaluation of extrapulmonary tuberculosis. It is a sensitive tool mostly used for the assessment of malignant disease; however, benign diseases and processes such as tissue repairs, infectious diseases, or inflammations (systemic vasculitis, granulomatous disease, postirradiation conditions, etc.) also show increased FDG uptake [7–10]. Therefore, FDG PET/CT is being used in extrapulmonary tuberculosis for precise identification of the activity and spread of the disease, which is crucial for further management as well as in follow-up of the therapy response (Fig. 7.1) [11].

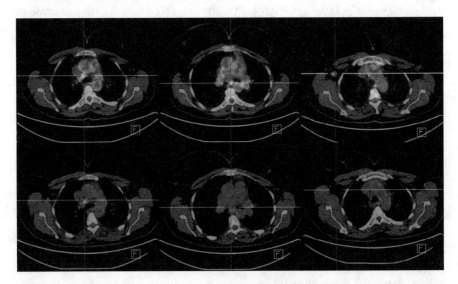

Fig. 7.1 FDG PET/CT in transversal plane: Evaluation of therapy response, before (upper images) and after therapy

7.1 Extrapulmonary Tuberculosis of the Lymph Nodes

Tuberculous lymphadenitis represents around 20–40% of extrapulmonary tuberculosis. As a nonspecific tracer, ^{18}F-FDG PET does not have the ability to differ malignancy, inflammation, or granulomatous diseases in the lymph nodes based on the standardized uptake value (SUV). SUV measurements could be high in tuberculosis as well as in malignant and other granulomatous lesions, with a significant overlap that limits their usefulness. Payabvash et al. studied the role of PET/CT in differentiating malignant from benign cervical lymph nodes in patients with head and neck cancer, showing that the SUVmax of $\geq$2.5 can be used in detection of malignant lymph nodes with 19% specificity, whereas a cutoff of $\geq$5.5 has 100% specificity [12]. However, in a study of Ding et al., an enlarged lymph node with SUVmax of 5.8 was also identified as tuberculosis [3].

Dual-time-point imaging is an additional technique used during routine ^{18}F-FDG PET/CT imaging to differentiate malignancy from underlying inflammatory or infectious diseases and contributes to the reduction of false-positive findings [13, 14]. Yamada et al. found that FDG uptake in inflammatory tissue increases until 60 min after the injection and then decreases gradually [15]. On the other hand, there is more and more evidence suggesting that tumor uptake of FDG increases for hours after the injection [16, 17].

Tuberculous granulomas are typically presented with an increased ^{18}F-FDG uptake (Fig. 9.3), so areas of active tuberculosis can be differentiated from old or inactive disease [18]. A study of Sathekge et al. showed that the lymph nodes responding to antituberculous treatment could be differentiated from the nonresponding ones using SUVmax cut-off value of 4.5 with a sensitivity of 95% and specificity of 85% [19].

In extrapulmonary tuberculosis, most commonly involved lymph nodes are cervical (Fig. 7.2) as well as suprascapular and to the lesser extent submandibular and periauricular. Cervical tuberculous lymphadenopathy, also known as "scrofula" or "king's evil," can be presented as a painless, mobile swelling. Infected superficial lymph nodes may also cause overlaying skin inflammation, which results in ulceration as a first manifestation. Sometimes, cervical adenopathy can lead to the upper airway obstruction by compressing trachea [20, 21].

Intrathoracic tuberculous lymphadenopathy (Fig. 7.3) includes hilar and/or mediastinal lymph nodes which may cause chest pain, dry cough, shortness of breath, dysphagia, etc. The incidence of conjoined pulmonary involvement deviates from 5% to 62% [22–24].

Abdominal lymphadenopathy can be localized or generalized (Figs. 7.4 and 7.5). Most commonly affected are periportal, peripancreatic, mesenteric, omental, and upper paraaortic lymph nodes. It can be asymptomatic, or it can cause nonspecific symptoms such as abdominal pain, abdominal distension, vomiting, diarrhea, and anorexia [25–27]. FDG PET/CT shows high false-positive rates in abdominal tuberculosis [28, 29], but the distribution pattern may help in distinguishing tuberculosis from carcinomatous dissemination [30].

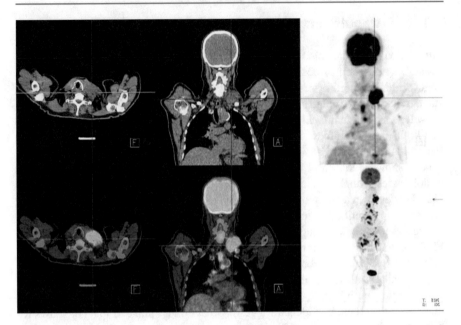

Fig. 7.2 CT and PET/CT in transversal and coronal plane, PET in coronal plane, and maximal intensity projection (MIP): A lymph node conglomerate with intense accumulation of FDG (SUVmax 22.3) in IV jugular group on the left side of the neck

Axillar and inguinal lymph nodes are also included in tuberculosis (Fig. 7.6), sometimes as the only manifestation [31, 32].

Caution should be taken in interpretation of the lymph node involvement in tuberculosis, while it could be misdiagnosed with lymphadenopathy caused by malignant diseases such as Hodgkin's and Non-Hodgkin's lymphoma, lymph node metastases, other granulomatous diseases including active sarcoidosis, or lymph node involvement in HIV-positive patients [3, 33–37]. In order to appropriately use PET/CT to distinguish an active tuberculous lesion from malignancy, especially in the lymph nodes, various other PET tracers have been investigated. Hara et al. compared ^{18}F-FDG and ^{11}C-choline uptake in cancer and tuberculous lymph nodes in their study, concluding that only cancer cells show high uptake with choline, and tuberculous lesions are hardly visualized [38]. In addition, dual-time-point imaging or double-phase techniques of FDG PET/CT have been suggested. However, histopathological verification is needed for definitive diagnosis and whole body FDG PET/CT scans provide an insight of the disease spread and accurate localization of the lymph nodes for biopsy based on SUVmax [39, 40].

7.2   Extrapulmonary Tuberculosis of Genitourinary Tract

Urogenital tuberculosis is a frequent location and accounts for 15–20% of all cases of extrapulmonary tuberculosis [5]. Approximately 75% of renal tuberculous involvement is unilateral with the most common finding being renal calcification.

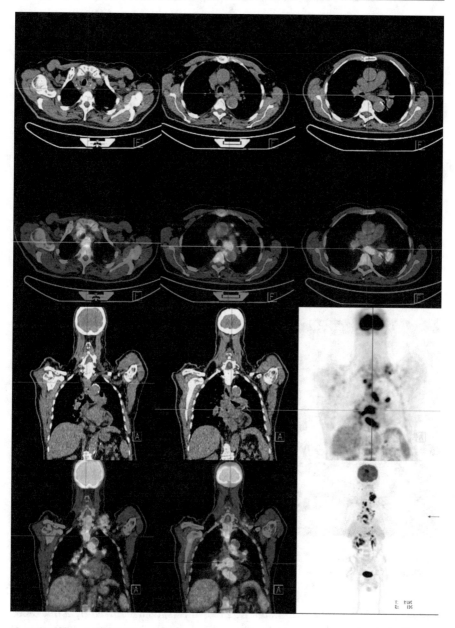

Fig. 7.3 CT and PET/CT in transversal and coronal plane, PET in coronal plane, and MIP: Enlarged paratracheal, paraoesophageal, aortopulmonary, subcarinal, hilar lymph nodes with an increased uptake of FDG (SUVmax 21.5)

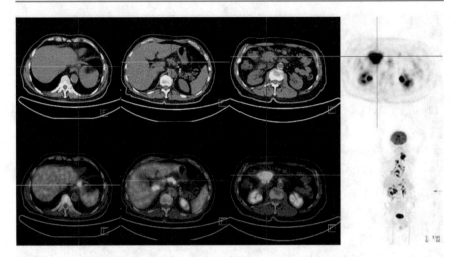

Fig. 7.4 CT, PET, and PET/CT in transversal plane and MIP: Enlarged hepatogastric, hepatoduodenal, mesenteric lymph nodes and in the liver hilum with an increased uptake of FDG (SUVmax 10.6)

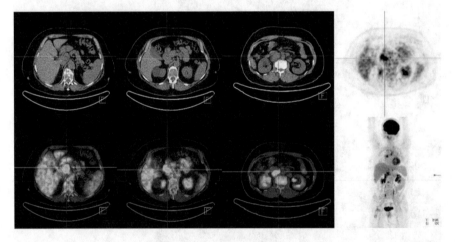

Fig. 7.5 CT, PET, and PET/CT in transversal plane and MIP: Increased uptake is shown in liver hilum, precaval, and paraaortic lymph nodes (SUVmax 9.2)

Almost 50% is conjoined with ureteric tuberculosis, characterized by a thickened ureteric wall and strictures in the distal third mostly [41]. Two morphological appearances are seen routinely: pyelonephritis or a pseudotumoural type presenting as single or multiple nodules. Gambhir et al. uncovered in their study tuberculous pyelonephritis using ^{18}F-FDG PET/CT and proved its role in evaluation of renal masses [42], while Subramanyam et al. emphasized the importance of ^{18}F-FDG PET/CT dual-time-point imaging in identifying renal metastatic deposits versus

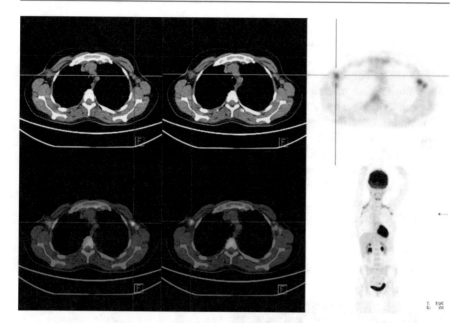

Fig. 7.6   CT, PET, and PET/CT in transversal plane and MIP: Enlarged axillary lymph nodes bilaterally with an increased uptake of FDG (SUVmax 4.6), as the only manifestation of tuberculosis

coexisting renal tuberculosis in their patient [43]. In fact, 2 h post-injection FDG showed partial clearance from the renal lesions (SUVmax of 4.2 vs. initial SUVmax of 6.2), which raised a suspicion of an infective pathology and false-positive finding was avoided. This proved that FDG PET/CT dual-time-point technique enhances the specificity in diagnosing infections. Even though different lesions of the urinary system can be detected on PET/CT as hotspots, high concentration of the excreted FDG in urine can mask FDG-avid lesions and limit image interpretation [44, 45].

Involvement of the genital organs occurs in 1.5% of females affected with tuberculosis, and almost always involves the fallopian tubes (94% of cases), usually causing bilateral salpingitis [46]. Sharma et al. showed in their study that ^{18}F-FDG PET/CT detection rates of tubo-ovarian masses were similar to those obtained with CT or MRI, but the characterization of adnexal masses was poorer [47]. Ovarian lesions may show moderate uptake on ^{18}F-FDG PET/CT with SUVmax 4.4, keeping in mind the possibility of physiological uterine and ovarian uptake [42]. Male involvement is confined to the seminal vesicles or prostate gland, with occasional calcifications (10% of cases). Prostatic tuberculosis can show high focal FDG uptake on PET/CT, which is often difficult to distinguish from malignancy such as prostatic adenocarcinoma [48], but ^{18}F-FDG PET may be helpful in characterizing prostatic tuberculosis and monitoring antituberculous treatment [49]. Physiological FDG uptake in testis must be taken into consideration while evaluating tuberculous involvement [50].

7.3   Extrapulmonary TB of Pleura, Peritoneum, and Pericardium

Tuberculous pleural effusion is the second most common form of extrapulmonary tuberculosis, often manifested as an acute illness (Fig. 7.7). It is usually unilateral and small to moderate in size, although massive effusion can occur [51]. FDG PET/ CT is an effective tool for differentiating between benign and malignant pleural diseases with sensitivity of 96.8% and specificity of 88.5% [52]. The most frequent sequela of pleural tuberculosis is a residual pleural thickening, which is why it can be mistaken with pleural mesothelioma on FDG PET. Yeh et al. reported a case of tuberculous pleuritis where abnormal distribution of FDG uptake mimicked malignant pleural mesothelioma [53]. In all cases of diffuse pleural thickening with intense FDG uptake, active tuberculosis should be considered in the differential diagnosis even when there are no subjective symptoms [54].

Peritoneal tuberculosis affects one-third of the patients and is one of the most common manifestations of abdominal tuberculosis. Malignant and benign disease

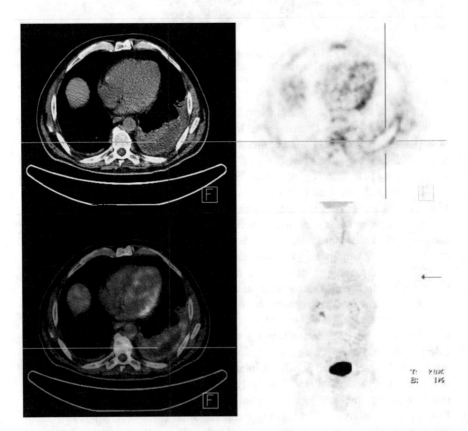

Fig. 7.7 CT, PET, and PET/CT in transversal plane and MIP: Diffuse and nonhomogeneous uptake of FDG in thickened pleura with pleural effusion in left hemithorax (SUVmax 3.2)

involving peritoneum can be manifested as various imaging patterns on FDG PET/CT [55]. An intense FDG activity in peritoneal tuberculous thickening can mimic peritoneal carcinomatosis [28, 56], where PET/CT can be a useful diagnostic tool for peritoneal biopsy [57]. In a study of Chen et al. some factors were significantly different between the patients with peritoneal thickening in tuberculosis and malignancy which included age, pattern of peritoneal thickening, and presence of ascites [58]. Significant difference in SUVmax was not found between malignant and benign peritoneal thickening. SUVmax was significantly higher in malignant than in nontuberculous benign peritoneal thickening, but the SUVmax of the thickened peritoneum was significantly higher in tuberculous than in nontuberculous benign cases. Tuberculous peritoneal thickening showed a hypermetabolic pattern, with SUVmax in the range of 1.7–8.6.

Cardiac tuberculosis is rare and generally involves the pericardium, accounting for only 0.5% of cases of extrapulmonary tuberculosis [59]. Usefulness of ^{18}F-FDG PET/CT in the detection of pericardial tuberculosis was assessed by Jiang et al., who proved that features like pericardial thickening and enhancement of FDG uptake, mediastinal lymph node enlargement, and their enhancement of FDG uptake may help in differentiation of pericardial and idiopathic pericarditis [60]. Also, mediastinal lymph nodes without hilar involvement may help to differentiate it from malignant pericardial disease [61]. FDG PET/CT can be a useful tool in evaluation of a therapy response to tuberculostatics in patients with pericarditis [62].

7.4 Abdominal Extrapulmonary TB: Hepatosplenic, Gastrointestinal, and Adrenal

Hepatosplenic involvement is commonly seen in patients with disseminated tuberculosis (Fig. 7.8). The pattern of FDG uptake varies, showing diffuse and focal uptake, followed by hepatosplenomegaly and lymph node involvement. CT images of PET/CT are helpful in characterizing the lesions morphologically and the use of intravenous contrast may increase the specificity of diagnosis in some instances, by demonstrating more accurately the presence of necrosis or typical focal lesions in the liver and spleen [44]. Also, hepatic tuberculosis can be manifested on PET/CT as a hepatic superscan with reduced physiological activity in the brain and heart mimicking lymphoma [63]. It is reported that diffuse hepatosplenic FDG uptake without focal anatomical lesions may be a predictor of tuberculosis after lymphoma in these organs [64]. PET/CT is helpful in detection of tuberculosis in cases of fever of unknown origin and when other imaging modalities are negative [65, 66].

Any part of the gastrointestinal tract can be affected by tuberculosis, from the esophagus to the anal canal, most commonly involved regions are distal ileum and caecum (Fig. 7.9). It may be presented as a bowel mass, indistinguishable from bowel cancer on routine imaging modalities, and may exhibit intense uptake on FDG PET imaging [67]. It can be difficult to distinguish multisite abdominal tuberculosis from malignancy even with ^{18}F-FDG PET/CT, when dual-time-point imaging is suggested [29]. Gastrointestinal tract, especially intestine and colon, is a site

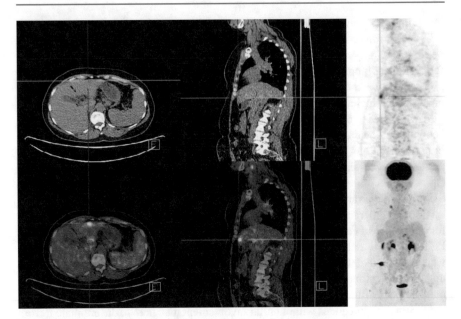

Fig. 7.8 CT, PET, and PET/CT in transversal, sagittal plane and MIP: Focally increased uptake of FDG in the left lobe of the liver (SUVmax 5.2)

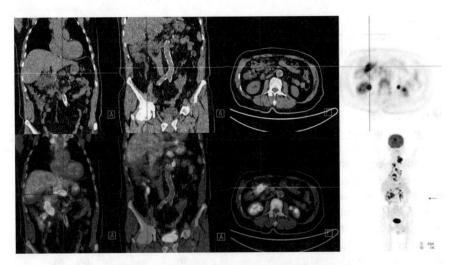

Fig. 7.9 CT, PET, and PET/CT in coronal, transversal plane and MIP: Focally increased uptake in the intestines (SUVmax 9.7), which could be mistaken with physiological finding

well known for physiologic accumulation of FDG, which can be a practical problem in the evaluation of PET images [68].

Adrenal tuberculosis is usually bilateral, with calcification on unenhanced CT and increased FDG uptake due to granulomatous formation [69, 70], which can be misdiagnosed for malignancy [71–73]. In a study of Yun et al., FDG PET showed excellent diagnostic performance in differentiating adrenal lesions detected on CT or MRI, with a sensitivity of 100%, specificity of 94%, and an accuracy of 96% [74]. Maurea et al. claim that abnormally increased FDG uptake in adrenal malignancies allows differentiation from benign lesions [75]. However, in another study of four patients with adrenal tuberculosis, ^{18}F-FDG PET/CT scan showed high uptake in bilateral tumors in two patients (SUVmax 12.3–19) which suggested malignancy, but in the other two patients ^{18}F-FDG PET/CT showed lower uptake with SUVmax 3.2 and 4.8 [76]. It is thought that this could have been the result of a lack of granulomatous inflammation due to the local suppressive effect of the steroids secreted in the adrenal cortex.

7.5   Extrapulmonary Tuberculosis of Musculoskeletal System

Musculoskeletal system is involved in only 1–3% of cases of tuberculosis, with parts most frequently affected including spinal column, pelvis, hip, and knee [59]. Approximately 50% of skeletal tuberculosis involves the spine, mostly lower thoracic and upper lumbar level. Tuberculous lesions are found to have increased FDG uptake in the active regions of granulomatous inflammation, with cold areas that represent necrotized tissue in spine [77]. SUVmax can be taken as a reliable marker for serial quantification of metabolic activity in spinal tuberculosis and useful for discrimination of residual and nonresidual infection after treatment [78, 79]. Unlike MR, FDG PET can be performed when there is an implant or an artifact at the examination site and it was superior in the identification of involved nodal basins compared to CT alone in a study of Zinn et al. [80].

In patients with FDG-avid bone lesions of unknown causes, granulomatous disease, such as tuberculosis and sarcoidosis, should be considered [81, 82]. Skeletal tuberculosis can mimic malignant lesion with its destruction of bones and increased FDG uptake on PET imaging (Fig. 7.10). Even though the diagnostic specificity of PET/CT in skeletal tuberculosis is not sufficient, it has proven to be a valuable modality for the identification of the most appropriate biopsy site for histopathological evaluation and diagnosis [79–83].

It has been reported that FDG PET has an outstanding potential to diagnose osteomyelitis. Excluding the diagnosis of chronic osteomyelitis is often difficult with noninvasive techniques, especially when bone anatomy and structures have been altered by trauma, surgery, or soft-tissue infection. In a study of Zhuang et al., FDG PET correctly diagnosed the presence and absence of chronic osteomyelitis in 20 out of 22 patients [84]. This study had a sensitivity of 100%, specificity of 87.5%, and accuracy of 90.9%. FDG PET is a highly effective imaging method to exclude osteomyelitis when a negative scan result is obtained, however, positive results can be caused not only by true osteomyelitis but also by inflammation in the bone or surrounding soft tissues as a result of other causes [85]. Schmitz et al. showed in their study that FGD PET is a very sensitive imaging modality in the detection of

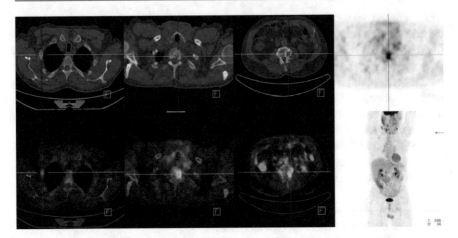

Fig. 7.10 CT, PET, and PET/CT in transversal plane and MIP: Osteolytic lesions in ribs and vertebrae with an increased uptake of FDG mimicking malignancy (vertebral SUVmax 6.4)

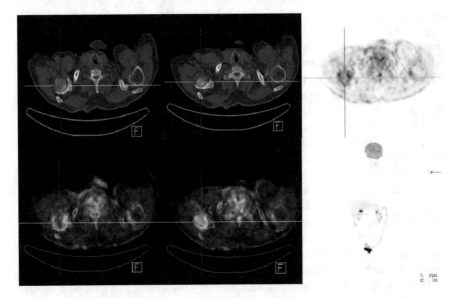

Fig. 7.11 CT, PET, and PET/CT in transversal plane and MIP: Increased and nonhomogeneous uptake of FDG in glenohumeral joint on the left side; histology confirmed tuberculous osteoarthritis

spondylodiscitis [86]. FDG PET was true positive in 12 patients, true negative in 3, and false positive in 1. SUVmax was 7.5 ± 3.8. Paravertebral soft tissue involvement can also be described in cases of spondylodiscitis.

Tuberculous arthritis is manifested typically as a monoarthritis affecting large weight-bearing joints (Figs. 7.11 and 7.12). The imaging findings are nonspecific and similar to those of other infectious and inflammatory arthritis [87]. In a study of

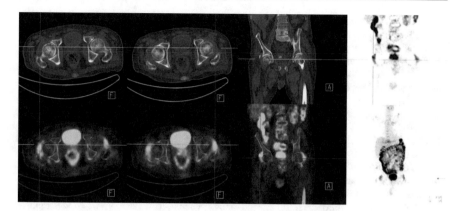

Fig. 7.12 CT, PET, and PET/CT in transversal, coronal plane and MIP: Diffuse uptake of FDG around femoral head bilaterally; histology confirmed tuberculous osteoarthritis

Wang et al., whole-body PET/CT scan revealed an intense FDG uptake in the left joint of the hip, which was subsequently confirmed by culture to be tuberculous osteoarthritis [88].

7.6   Conclusion

The role of ^{18}F-FDG PET/CT is important in the detection, assessment of activity, and the extent of extrapulmonary tuberculosis. ^{18}F-FDG PET detects more tuberculous lesions than CT, and it is used in cases when other imaging modalities are negative. It is of great value in monitoring response to antituberculosis treatment by separating active from inactive disease with high sensitivity, as the degree of FDG uptake is equivalent to the severity of infection. There is an overlap in SUVmax values of tuberculous and inflammatory or malignant lesions on ^{18}F-FDG PET, which is a limitation factor, however whole-body FDG PET/CT scans provide an insight into the disease spread and accurate localization of the lesions for biopsy, based on SUVmax. Dual-time-point technique increases the specificity in diagnosing infections versus malignancy.

References

1. World Health Organization. Definitions and reporting framework for tuberculosis: 2013 revision (updated December 2014). Geneva: World Health Organization; 2013.
2. Harisinghani MG, McLoud TC, Shepard JO, Ko JP, Shroff MM, Mueller PR. Tuberculosis from head to toe. Radiographics. 2000;20:449–70. https://doi.org/10.1148/radiographics.20.2.g00mc12449.
3. Ding RL, Cao HY, Hu Y, Shang CL, Xie F, Zhang ZH, Wen QL. Lymph node tuberculosis mimicking malignancy on 18F-FDG PET/CT in two patients: a case report. Exp Ther Med. 2017;13:3369–73. https://doi.org/10.3892/etm.2017.4421.

4. Palacios Vivar DE, Torres Cruz YJ, Villasana JEM. Diagnosis of extra-pulmonary tuberculosis: systematic analysis of literature and study of seven cases in the cervicofacial region. Revista Odontológica Mexicana. 2016;20:258–64.
5. Engin G, Acunaş B, Acunaş G, Tunaci M. Imaging of extrapulmonary tuberculosis. Radiographics. 2000;20:471–88. https://doi.org/10.1148/radiographics.20.2.g00mc07471.
6. Watkins RE, Brennan R, Plant AJ. Tuberculin reactivity and the risk of tuberculosis: a review. Int J Tuberc Lung Dis. 2000;4:895–903. https://doi.org/10.1016/S0218-0014(00)00057-X.
7. Rosenbaum SJ, Lind T, Antoch G, Bockisch A. False-positive FDG PET uptake—the role of PET/CT. Eur Radiol. 2006;16:1054–65. https://doi.org/10.1007/s00330-005-0088-y.
8. Chang JM, Lee HJ, Goo JM, Lee HY, Lee JJ, Chung JK, Im JG. False positive and false negative FDG-PET scans in various thoracic diseases. Korean J Radiol. 2006;7:57–69. https://doi.org/10.3348/kjr.2006.7.1.57.
9. Ichiya Y, Kuwabara Y, Sasaki M, Yoshida T, Akashi Y, Murayama S, et al. FDG-PET in infectious lesions: the detection and assessment of lesion activity. Ann Nucl Med. 1996;10:185–91.
10. Sobic-Saranovic D, Grozdic I, Videnovic-Ivanov J, Vucinic-Mihailovic V, Artiko V, Saranovic DJ, et al. The utility of 18F-fluoro-deoxy-glucose PET/CT for diagnosis and adjustment of therapy in patients with active chronic sarcoidosis. J Nucl Med. 2012;53:1543–9. https://doi.org/10.2967/jnumed.112.104380.
11. Sathekge M, Maes A, Van de Wiele C. FDG-PET imaging in HIV infection and tuberculosis. Semin Nucl Med. 2013;43:349–66. https://doi.org/10.1053/j.semnuclmed.2013.04.008.
12. Payabvash S, Meric K, Cayci Z. Differentiation of benign from malignant cervical lymph nodes in patients with head and neck cancer using PET/CT imaging. Clin Imaging. 2016;40:101–5. https://doi.org/10.1016/j.clinimag.2015.09.001.
13. Kubota K, Itoh M, Ozaki K, Ono S, Tashiro M, Yamaguchi K, et al. Advantage of delayed whole-body FDG-PET imaging for tumour detection. Eur J Nucl Med. 2001;28:696–703. https://doi.org/10.1007/s002590100537.
14. Zhuang H, Pourdehnad M, Lambright ES. Dual time point 18F-FDG PET imaging for differentiating malignant from inflammatory processes. J Nucl Med. 2001;42:1412–7.
15. Yamada S, Kubota K, Kubota R, Ido T, Tamahashi N. High accumulation of fluorine-18-fluorodeoxyglucose in turpentine-induced inflammatory tissue. J Nucl Med. 1995;36:1301–6.
16. Hamberg LM, Hunter GJ, Alpert NM, Choi NC, Babich JW, Fischman AJ. The dose uptake ratio as an index of glucose metabolism: useful parameter or oversimplification? J Nucl Med. 1994;35:1308–12.
17. Lodge MA, Lucas JD, Marsden PK, Cronin BF, O'Doherty MJ, Smith MA. A PET study of 18FDG uptake in soft tissue masses. Eur J Nucl Med. 1999;26:22–30. https://doi.org/10.1007/s002590050355.
18. Vorster M, Sathekge MM, Bomanji J. Advances in imaging of tuberculosis: the role of 18F-FDG PET and PET/CT. Curr Opin Pulm Med. 2014;20:287–93. https://doi.org/10.1097/MCP.0000000000000043.
19. Sathekge M, Maes A, D'Asseler Y, Vorster M, Gongxeka H, Van de Wiele C. Tuberculous lymphadenitis: FDG PET and CT findings in responsive and nonresponsive disease. Eur J Nucl Med Mol Imaging. 2012;39:1184–90. https://doi.org/10.1007/s00259-012-2115-y.
20. Moulis G, Martin-Blondel G. Scrofula, the king's evil. Can Med Assoc J. 2012;184:1061. https://doi.org/10.1503/cmaj.111519.
21. Gupta PR. Difficulties in managing lymph node tuberculosis. Lung India. 2004;21:50–3. https://doi.org/10.14744/nci.2016.20982.
22. Venkateswaran RV, Barron DJ, Brawn WJ, Clarke JR, Desai M, Samuel M, Parikh DH. A forgotten old disease: mediastinal tuberculous lymphadenitis in children. Eur J Cardiothorac Surg. 2005;27:401–4. https://doi.org/10.1016/j.ejcts.2004.12.014.
23. Xiong L, Mao X, Li C, Liu Z, Zhang Z. Posterior mediastinal tuberculous lymphadenitis with dysphagia as the main symptom: a case report and literature review. J Thorac Dis. 2013;5:E189–94. https://doi.org/10.3978/j.issn.2072-1439.2013.09.03.
24. Iyengar KB, Udyavara Kudru C, Kaniyoor Nagiri S, Rao ACK. Tuberculous mediastinal lymphadenopathy in an adult. BMJ Case Rep. 2014;2014. https://doi.org/10.1136/bcr-2013-200718.

25. Ramesh J, Banait GS, Ormerod LP. Abdominal tuberculosis in a district general hospital: a retrospective review of 86 cases. QJM. 2008;101:189–95. https://doi.org/10.1093/qjmed/hcm125.
26. Arvind M, Shubham A, Shilpa. Abdominal lymphadenopathy—tuberculosis mimicking classy clinicoradiological features of Hodgkin's disease. JAMA. 2016;5:43–5. https://doi.org/10.5958/2319-4324.2016.00010.9.
27. Yang ZG, Min PQ, Sone S, He ZY, Liao ZY, Zhou XP, et al. Tuberculosis versus lymphomas in the abdominal lymph nodes: evaluation with contrast-enhanced CT. AJR. 1999;172:619–23. https://doi.org/10.2214/ajr.172.3.10063847.
28. Shimamoto H, Hamada K, Higuchi I, Tsujihata M, Nonomura N, Tomita Y, et al. Abdominal tuberculosis: peritoneal involvement shown by F-18 FDG PET. Clin Nucl Med. 2007;32:716–8. https://doi.org/10.1097/RLU.0b013e318123f813.
29. Tian G, Xiao Y, Chen B, Guan H, Deng QY. Multi-site abdominal tuberculosis mimics malignancy on 18F-FDG PET/CT: report of three cases. World J Gastroenterol. 2010;16:4237–42. https://doi.org/10.3748/wjg.v16.i33.4237.
30. Jeffry L, Kerrou K, Camatte S, Lelievre L, Metzger U, Robin F, et al. Peritoneal tuberculosis revealed by carcinomatosis on CT scan and uptake at FDG-PET. BJOG. 2003;110:1129–31. https://doi.org/10.1111/j.1471-0528.2003.03070.x.
31. Hui L, Qiang L. Tuberculous lymphadenitis in the left axillary misdiagnosed as metastasis: a case report and review of literature. Radiol Infect Dis. 2017;4:38–44. https://doi.org/10.1016/j.jrid.2016.06.002.
32. Lawee D. Primary tuberculous inguinal lymphadenitis. Can Med Assoc J. 1969;100:34–6.
33. Sathekge M, Maes A, Kgomo M, Stoltz A, Van de Wiele C. Use of 18F-FDG PET to predict response to first-line tuberculostatics in HIV-associated tuberculosis. J Nucl Med. 2011;52:880–5. https://doi.org/10.2967/jnumed.110.083709.
34. Sathekge M, Maes A, Kgomo M, Pottel H, Stolz A, Van De Wiele C. FDG uptake in lymphnodes of HIV+ and tuberculosis patients: implications for cancer staging. J Nucl Med Mol Imaging. 2010;54:698–703.
35. Huber H, Lang D, Fellner F, Lamprecht B, Gabriel M. Tuberculosis and Sarcoidosis imaging in 18F-FDG-PET/CT: consistencies and inconsistencies. J Nucl Med. 2018;59:1599.
36. Treglia G, Annunziata S, Sobic-Saranovic D, Bertagna F, Caldarella C, Giovanella L. The role of 18F-FDG PET and PET/CT in patients with sarcoidosis: an update and evidence-based review. Acad Radiol. 2014;21:675–84. https://doi.org/10.1016/j.acra.2014.01.008.
37. Sobic-Saranovic D, Artiko V. Obradovic V.FDG PET imaging in sarcoidosis. Semin Nucl Med. 2013;43:404–11.
38. Hara T, Kosaka N, Suzuki T, Kudo K, Nino H. Uptake rates of 18F-fluorodeoxyglucose and 11C-choline in lung cancer and pulmonary tuberculosis: a positron emission tomography study. Chest. 2003;124:893–901. https://doi.org/10.1378/chest.124.3.893.
39. Castaigne C, Garcia C, Flamen P. Tuberculosis on FDG PET-CT: the great imitator. J Nucl Med. 2014;55:1969.
40. Bhattacharya A, Agrawal KL, Kashyap R, Manohar K, Mittal B, Varma SC, et al. Coexisting tuberculosis and non-Hodgkin's lymphoma on 18F-Fluorodeoxyglucose PET-CT. JPMER. 2012;46:49–50. https://doi.org/10.5005/jp-journals-10028-1012.
41. Zissin R, Gayer G, Chowers M, Shapiro-Feinberg M, Kots E, Hertz M. Computerized tomography findings of abdominal tuberculosis: report of 19 cases. Isr Med Assoc J. 2001;3:414–8.
42. Gambhir S, Ravina M, Rangan K, Dixit M, Barai S, Bomanji J, et al. Imaging in extrapulmonary tuberculosis. Int J Infect Dis. 2017;56:237–47. https://doi.org/10.1016/j.ijid.2016.11.003.
43. Subramanyam P, Palaniswamy SS. Dual time point (18)F-FDG PET/CT imaging identifies bilateral renal tuberculosis in an Immunocompromised patient with an unknown primary malignancy. Infect Chemother. 2015;47:117–9. https://doi.org/10.3947/ic.2015.47.2.117.
44. Harkirat S, Anana SS, Indrajit LK, Dash AK. Pictorial essay: PET/CT in tuberculosis. Indian J Radiol Imaging. 2008;18:141–7. https://doi.org/10.4103/0971-3026.40299.
45. Kochhar R, Brown RK, Wong CO, Dunnick NR, Frey KA, Manoharan P. Role of FDG PET/CT in imaging of renal lesions. J Med Imag Radiat Oncol. 2010;54:347–57. https://doi.org/10.1111/j.1754-9485.2010.02181.x.

46. Wang LJ, Wong YC, Chen CJ, Lim KE. CT features of genitourinary tuberculosis. J Comput Assist Tomogr. 1997;21:254–8.

47. Sharma JB, Karmakar D, Kumar R, Shamim SA, Kumar S, Singh N, et al. Comparison of PET/CT with other imaging modalities in women with genital tuberculosis. Int J Gynaecol Obstet. 2012;118:123–8. https://doi.org/10.1016/j.ijgo.2012.02.020.

48. Kadihasanoglu M, Yildiz T, Atahan S, Ausmus A, Atahan O. 18F-flouro-2-deoxyglucose positron emission tomography/computed tomography imaging of solitary prostatic and pulmonary tuberculosis mimicking metastatic prostate cancer. J Cancer Res Ther. 2015;11:663. https://doi.org/10.4103/0973-1482.143354.

49. Lee G, Lee JH, Park SG. F-18 FDG PET/CT imaging of solitary genital tuberculosis mimicking recurrent lymphoma. Clin Nucl Med. 2011;36:315–6. https://doi.org/10.1097/RLU.0b013e31820aa033.

50. Agarwal K, Behera A, Kumar R, Bal C. 18F-Fluorodeoxyglucose-positron emission tomography/ computed tomography in tuberculosis: Spectrum of manifestations. Indian J Nucl Med. 2017;32:316–21. https://doi.org/10.4103/ijnm.IJNM_29_17.

51. Zhai K, Lu Y, Shi HZ. Tuberculous pleural effusion. J Thorac Dis. 2016;8:E486. https://doi.org/10.21037/jtd.2016.05.87.

52. Duysinx B, Nguyen D, Louis R, Cataldo D, Belhocine T, Bartsch P, Bury T. Evaluation of pleural disease with 18-fluorodeoxyglucose positron emission tomography imaging. Chest. 2004;125:489–93. https://doi.org/10.1378/chest.125.2.489.

53. Yeh CL, Chen LK, Chen SW, Chen YK. Abnormal FDG PET imaging in tuberculosis appearing like mesothelioma: anatomic delineation by CT can aid in differential diagnosis. Clin Nucl Med. 2009;34:815–7. https://doi.org/10.1097/RLU.0b013e3181b81e09.

54. Shinohara T, Shiota N, Kume M, Hamada N, Naruse K, Ogushi F. Asymptomatic primary tuberculous pleurisy with intense 18-fluorodeoxyglucose uptake mimicking malignant mesothelioma. BMC Infect Dis. 2013;13:1. https://doi.org/10.1186/1471-2334-13-12.

55. Anthony MP, Khong PL, Zhang J. Spectrum of (18)F-FDG PET/CT appearances in peritoneal disease. AJR Am J Roentgenol. 2009;193:W523–9. https://doi.org/10.2214/AJR.09.2936.

56. Takalkar AM, Bruno GL, Reddy M, Lilien DL. Intense FDG activity in peritoneal tuberculosis mimics peritoneal carcinomatosis. Clin Nucl Med. 2007;32:244–6. https://doi.org/10.1097/01.rlu.0000255239.04475.c2.

57. Turlakow A, Yeung HW, Salmon AS, Macapinlac HA, Larson SM. Peritoneal carcinomatosis: role of (18)F-FDG PET. J Nucl Med. 2003;44:1407–12.

58. Chen R, Chen Y, Liu L, Zhou X, Liu J, Huang G. The role of ^{18}F-FDG PET/CT in the evaluation of peritoneal thickening of undetermined origin. Medicine (Baltimore). 2016;95:e3023. https://doi.org/10.1097/MD.0000000000003023.

59. Burrill J, Williams CJ, Bain G, Conder G, Hine AL, Misra R. Tuberculosis: a radiologic review. Radiographics. 2007;27:1255–73. https://doi.org/10.1148/rg.275065176.

60. Jiang Z, Xu X, Sun J, Liu B, Ding C, Li T. Usefulness of 18F-FDG PET/CT for the diagnosis of Tuberculous pericarditis. J Med Imaging Health Inform. 2017;7:460–3. https://doi.org/10.1166/jmihi.2017.1775.

61. Dong A, Dong H, Wang Y, Cheng C, Zuo C, Lu J. (18)F-FDG PET/CT in differentiating acute tuberculous from idiopathic pericarditis: preliminary study. Clin Nucl Med. 2013;38:e160–5. https://doi.org/10.1097/RLU.0b013e31827a2537.

62. Ozmen O, Koksal D, Ozcan A, Tatci E, Gokcek A. Decreased metabolic uptake in tuberculous pericarditis indicating response to antituberculosis therapy on FDG PET/CT. Clin Nucl Med. 2014;39:917–9. https://doi.org/10.1097/RLU.0000000000000443.

63. Man-Wong S, Yuen H, Ahuja AT. Hepatic tuberculosis: a rare cause of fluorodeoxyglucose hepatic superscan with background suppression on positron emission tomography. Singap Med J. 2014;55:e101–3. https://doi.org/10.11622/smedj.2013237.

64. Jeong YJ, Sohn MH, Lim ST, Kim DW, Jeong HJ, Chung MJ, et al. 'Hot liver' on 18F-FDG PET/CT imaging in a patient with hepatosplenic tuberculosis. Eur J Nucl Med Mol Imaging. 2010;37:1618–9. https://doi.org/10.1007/s00259-010-1477-2.

65. Yu HY, Sheng JF. Liver tuberculosis presenting as an uncommon cause of pyrexia of unknown origin: positron emission tomography/computed tomography identifies the correct site for biopsy. Med Princ Pract. 2014;23:577–9. https://doi.org/10.1159/000357869.
66. Anuradha R, Govindarajan M, Sharanabasappa G, Swarna S. Isolated splenic tuberculosis detected only on FDG-PET. BJR Case Rep. 2017;3:3. https://doi.org/10.1259/bjrcr.20150238.
67. Wang HY, Lin WY. Jejunal tuberculosis: incidental finding on an FDG-PET scan. Kaohsiung J Med Sci. 2006;22:34–8. https://doi.org/10.1016/S1607-551X(09)70218-9.
68. Kim SK, Chung JK, Kim BT, Kim SJ, Jeong JM, Lee DS, Lee MC. Relationship between gastrointestinal F-18-fluorodeoxyglucose accumulation and gastrointestinal symptoms in whole-body PET. Clin Positron Imaging. 1999;2:273–9. https://doi.org/10.1016/S1095-0397(99)00030-8.
69. Dong A, Cui Y, Wang Y, Zuo C, Bai Y. 18F-FDG PET/CT of adrenal lesions. AJR. 2014;203:245–52. https://doi.org/10.2214/ajr.13.11793.
70. Roudaut N, Malecot M, Dupont E, Boussion N, Visvikis D, Doucet L, et al. Adrenal tuberculosis revealed by FDG PET. Clin Nucl Med. 2008;33:821–3. https://doi.org/10.1097/RLU.0b013e318187ee60.
71. Wang L, Yang J. Tuberculous Addison's disease mimics malignancy in FDG-PET images. Intern Med. 2008;47:1755–6. https://doi.org/10.2169/internalmedicine.47.1348.
72. Yoon Y, Sung K, Yoon PY, OhDae T, Jung C. Adrenal tuberculosis mimicking a malignancy by direct hepatic invasion: emphasis on adrenohepatic fusion as the potential route. Clin Imaging. 2015;39:911–3. https://doi.org/10.1016/j.clinimag.2015.04.019.
73. Gorla R, Gupta K, Sood A, Biswal CK, Bhansali A, Mittal BR. Adrenal tuberculosis masquerading as disseminated malignancy: a pitfall of 18F-FDG PET/CT imaging. Rev Esp Med Nucl Imagen Mol (English Edition). 2016;35:257–9. https://doi.org/10.1016/j.remn.2015.11.008.
74. Yun M, Kim W, Alnafisi N, Lacorte L, Jang S, Alavi A. 18F-FDG PET in characterizing adrenal lesions detected on CT or MRI. J Nucl Med. 2001;42:1795–9.
75. Maurea S, Mainolfi C, Bazzicalupo L, Panico MR, Imparato C, Alfano B, et al. Imaging of adrenal tumors using FDG PET: comparison of benign and malignant lesions. AJR. 1999;173:25–9. https://doi.org/10.2214/ajr.173.1.10397094.
76. Kunikowska J, Matyskiel R, Toutounchi S, Grabowska-Derlatka L, Koperski L, Królicki L. What parameters from 18F-FDG PET/CT are useful in evaluation of adrenal lesions? Eur J Nucl Med Mol Imaging. 2014;41:2273–80. https://doi.org/10.1007/s00259-014-2844-1.
77. James SL, Davies AM. Imaging of infectious spinal disorders in children and adults. Eur J Radiol. 2006;58:27–40. https://doi.org/10.1016/j.ejrad.2005.12.002.
78. Dureja S, Sen IB, Acharya S. Potential role of F18 FDG PET-CT as an imaging biomarker for the noninvasive evaluation in uncomplicated skeletal tuberculosis: a prospective clinical observational study. Eur Spine J. 2014;23:2449–54. https://doi.org/10.1007/s00586-014-3483-8.
79. Cho YS, Chung DR, Lee EJ, Kim BT, Lee KH. 18F-FDG PET/CT in a case of multifocal skeletal tuberculosis without pulmonary disease and potential role for monitoring treatment response. Clin Nucl Med. 2014;39:980–3. https://doi.org/10.1097/RLU.0000000000000363.
80. Zinn C, Vorster M, Sathekge MM. Spinal tuberculosis evaluated by means of 18F-FDG PET/CT: pilot study. Open Nucl Med J. 2014;6:6–11. https://doi.org/10.2174/1876388X01406010006.
81. Grozdic Milojevic I, Sobic-Saranovic D, Videnovic-Ivanov J, Saranovic D, Odalovic S, Artiko V. FDG PET/CT in bone sarcoidosis. Sarcoidosis Vasc Diffuse Lung Dis. 2016;33:66–74.
82. Huang Z, Guan Y, Zuo C. PET/CT imaging of skeletal tuberculosis with FDG-avid lesions. J Nucl Med. 2013;54:1979.
83. Selçuk NA, Fenercioğlu A, Selçuk HH, Uluçay C, Yencilek E. Multifoci bone tuberculosis and lymphadenitis in mediastinum mimics malignancy on FDG-PET/CT: a case report. Mol Imaging Radionucl Ther. 2014;23:39–42. https://doi.org/10.4274/Mirt.145.
84. Zhuang H, Duarte PS, Pourdehand M, Shnier D, Alavi A. Exclusion of chronic osteomyelitis with F-18 fluorodeoxyglucose positron emission tomographic imaging. Clin Nucl Med. 2000;25:281–4. https://doi.org/10.1097/00003072-200004000-00009.

85. Kim SJ, Kim IJ, Suh KT, Kim YK, Lee JS. Prediction of residual disease of spine infection using F-18 FDG PET/CT. Spine (Phila Pa 1976). 2009;34:2424–30. https://doi.org/10.1097/BRS.0b013e3181b1fd33.
86. Schmitz A, Risse JH, Grünwald F, Gassel F, Biersack HJ, Schmitt O. Fluorine-18 fluorodeoxyglucose positron emission tomography findings in spondylodiscitis: preliminary results. Eur Spine J. 2001;10:534–9. https://doi.org/10.1007/s005860100339.
87. Berney S, Goldstein M, Bishko F. Clinical and diagnostic features of tuberculous arthritis. Am J Med. 1972;53:36–42. https://doi.org/10.1016/0002-9343(72)90113-1.
88. Wang JH, Chi CY, Lin KH, Ho MW, Kao CH. Tuberculous arthritis-unexpected extrapulmonary tuberculosis detected by FDG PET/CT. Clin Nucl Med. 2013;38:e93–4. https://doi.org/10.1097/RLU.0b013e318252d32e.

FDG PET in TB and HIV

8

T. M. G. Boshomane and Mike Sathekge

Contents

8.1 Introduction

Tuberculosis (TB) and human immunodeficiency virus (HIV) coinfection remains an important cause of morbidity and mortality burdens worldwide. The 2018 global report from the World Health Organization (WHO) reported the incidence burden as 10 million cases (5.8 million male, 3.2 million females, and one million children) with TB as the leading infectious disease cause of mortality in the world, with 1.6

T. M. G. Boshomane (✉) · M. Sathekge
Department of Nuclear Medicine, University of Pretoria & Steve Biko Academic Hospital, Pretoria, South Africa
e-mail: mike.sathekge@up.ac.za

© Springer Nature Switzerland AG 2020
D. Sobic Saranovic et al. (eds.), *PET/CT in Tuberculosis*, Clinicians' Guides to Radionuclide Hybrid Imaging, https://doi.org/10.1007/978-3-030-47009-8_8

million deaths occurring in 2017; this includes 0.3 million deaths among those with HIV coinfection [1–3].

TB and HIV are infections that are receiving global attention and can affect multiple organ systems. TB can occur in isolation or as a coinfection to HIV as an opportunistic infection (OI). Although the incidence of TB and HIV has been decreasing since 2000, these infectious diseases remain an important sustainable development goal (SDG).

The number of people living with HIV is growing due to the advent of antiretroviral therapy (ART); however, there is an unexpected increase in the resistance strains of TB and HIV. A growing population of patients are also presenting to healthcare centers requiring diagnostic techniques that are more accurate and less invasive.

Radionuclide imaging has been shown to be beneficial and to impact management in the oncology setting (e.g., lymphomas) and in benign settings (e.g., spondylodiskitis). Positron emission tomography (PET) has also been shown to be successful in numerous clinical scenarios, that is, staging, therapy evaluation/monitoring, detection of biopsy sites, and in fevers of unknown origin (FUO). The utility has been mainly demonstrated with fluorine-18 2-fluoro-2-deoxy-D-glucose (^{18}F-FDG, a sugar analogue) due to its availability and favorable physical characteristics (production and decay). FDG is transported into activated cells via glucose transporters that are activated during infection/inflammation. PET imaging with this radiopharmaceutical offers high-resolution imaging and precise localization.

In TB and HIV, PET imaging with ^{18}F-FDG has not yet been widely incorporated in routine clinical practice even though the sensitivity has been shown to be superior to conventional imaging tests in certain instances (e.g., spinal infections).

8.2   Pathophysiology of Tuberculosis

Mycobacterium tuberculosis is the bacterium responsible for pulmonary and extrapulmonary tuberculosis (EPTB) (Fig. 8.1) [4]. Pulmonary TB is present in the majority of cases, that is, >80%. However, the TB bacterium can affect any system in the body (CNS, cardiac, gastrointestinal, skeletal, ocular, and the genitourinary) [5]; TB outside the pulmonary system is termed extrapulmonary tuberculosis.

8.3   Pathophysiology of HIV

Infection and transmission of HIV occurs mainly through blood and the exposed/unprotected mucosal linings. HIV infects (with gp120 receptors), binds to T-cells that mainly express CD4 receptors (which are of lymphoid origin), and spreads to multiple organs. The virus can be detected in several organs systems (e.g., CNS, gastric-associated lymphoid tissue (GALT), pulmonary, genitalia, and the

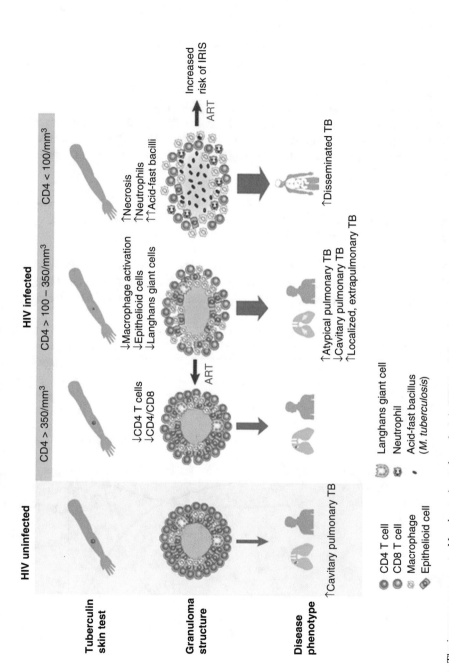

Fig. 8.1 The immune response to *Mycobacterium tuberculosis* in HIV-1-coinfected persons (Esmail H, Riou C, Bruyn ED, Lai RP, Harley YXR Meintjes G, Wilkinson KA, Wilkinson RJ. Annu Rev. Immunol. 2018;36:603–638 [4])

hemopoietic system); early and late clinical presentations have been described following infection (Fig. 8.2) [6]. CD4+ T-cells can also be found in the macrophages but are mainly found in the paracortex of the lymph nodes. Patients with HIV infection can present with a fever, rashes, and lymphadenopathy [7].

The natural history of HIV has three stages:

- Stage 1—Infection
- Stage 2—Dormancy/latency
- Stage 3—AIDS (acquired immunodeficiency syndrome)

More women than men have been documented to bear the worst brunt of HIV. Sathekge et al. have extensively demonstrated the utility of FDG PET in HIV-associated cancers (e.g., cervical, Kaposi's sarcoma (KS), breast and anal cancer, etc.) [8].

8.4   The Immune Response to *Mycobacterium tuberculosis* in HIV-1-Coinfected Persons

HIV-infected persons are 20–30 times more likely to develop TB than HIV-uninfected persons, who have only a 5–10% chance of developing active TB in their lifetime [9]. Furthermore, the leading cause of death in HIV-1-infected

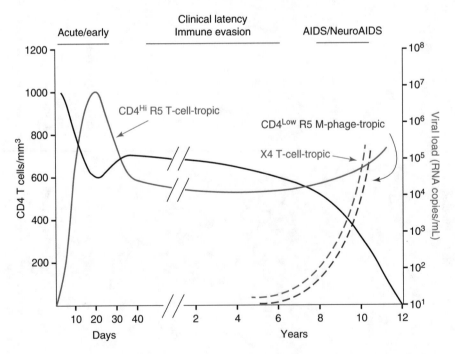

Fig. 8.2 Temporal relationship of CD4+ T-cells and HIV-1 infection. Adapted from Swanstrom et al.

people is tuberculosis. The impact of HIV-1 on tuberculosis alters the clinical presentation and makes it more difficult to diagnose, more complicated to treat, and results in a worse outcome. The risk of tuberculosis begins to increase within the first year of HIV-1 infection (in contrast to traditional opportunistic infections) and continues to increase as CD4+ T-cell depletion worsens, and it is incompletely reversed by effective antiretroviral therapy (ART) [4, 9]. This unusual feature of *M. tuberculosis* as an opportunist pathogen highlights wider immune deficits encompassing phagocyte function, antigen presentation, cytokine production, innate lymphocyte function, and B-cell and CD8+ T-cell function (See Fig. 8.2).

8.5 FDG PET and Fever of Unknown Origin (FUO)

Fever of unknown origin (FUO) is a complex and challenging clinical condition defined by persistent fever >38.3 °C, for >3 weeks, with no other confirmed diagnosis. Upon workup, the etiology has been found to be due to malignancy, inflammation (e.g. vasculitides), or infection, in which tuberculosis has been found to be contributory in ~20% of the cases [3, 10–13].Though other imaging techniques have been traditionally used to investigate FUO (e.g., X-ray, CT, and single-positron emission tomography (SPET)), imaging with ^{18}F-FDG PET has been shown to be useful.

^{18}F-FDG PET imaging has also been demonstrated to be a useful tool in HIV-negative and HIV-infected patients who are being worked up for FUO with no loss in interpretation confidence in patients with a high viral load [13].

8.6 Miliary TB

It is estimated that 1–2% of TB can be miliary. Miliary TB is defined as a lympho-hematogenous spread of the acid-fast bacilli; the typically pattern on radiology is the "millet seed" pattern. ^{18}F-FDG PET has been found useful in the detection of active lesions in the lungs and in other system (See Fig. 8.3) [10].

8.7 TB and HIV Lymphadenitis

The lymphatic system is an important host defense barrier and is involved primarily during infections and malignancy as a reservoir site [7].

In TB and HIV, the imaging findings have been described as typically symmetrical and reflect acute involvement in the cervical, axillary, and then to progress distally when the disease is in its chronic phase (See Fig. 8.4).

Fig. 8.3 Maximum
intensity projection of a
whole-body ^{18}F-FDG PET
in a patient diagnosed with
sputum-positive (acid-fast
bacilli) miliary tuberculosis

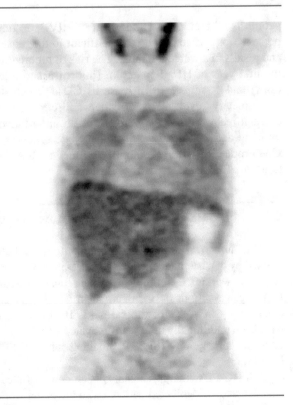

8.8   Cardiovascular System

The role of vascular inflammation has been receiving increasing attention as the
population of the elderly and those living with HIV rises. Stroke (CVI) and myocardial infarction (MI) risk increases by twofold in the setting of HIV infection [5, 14].

In regard to PET imaging with FDG, the role of HIV infection presenting as a
possible risk factor in patients with a low Framingham score, Subramanian et al.
have concluded that vascular inflammation increases in patients with HIV and thus
poses as a risk factor for coronary artery disease [15].

The value and role of FDG PET modality in diagnosing TB pericardial involvement in patients with and without HIV is evolving, as the pathogenesis of pericarditis is still being gradually understood. At present ^{18}F-FDG PET image findings are
nonspecific for pericarditis but may assist in excluding concurrent diseases [16–18].

8.9   Skeletal Infection

Palestro et al. [19–21] have documented the value of ^{18}F-FDG PET over other radionuclide imaging techniques in vertebral infections and in the immune-compromised
patients (e.g., HIV-infected populations), in endemic regions. *Mycobacterium
tuberculosis* remains an important cause of vertebral osteomyelitis. The role of [18]F-
FDG PET in patients with pedal osteomyelitis has not been fully established.

Fig. 8.4 Maximum intensity projection (MIP) image of an ^{18}F-FDG PET in a 26-year-old female infected with HIV and TB involving mediastinal nodes, lungs, abdominal lymphadenitis, and spleen

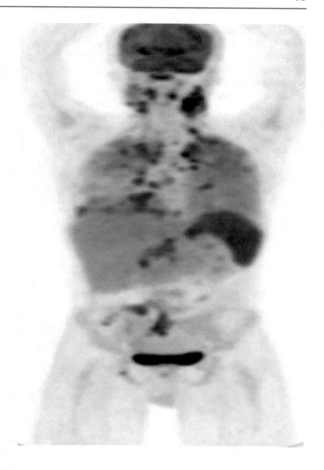

8.10   Urogenital TB

Urogenital TB accounts for ~1% cases of TB and < 6% of EPTB. Lee et al. [22] have reported an isolated case of genital TB using ^{18}F-FDG PET. The rarity and lack of standard defining of urogenital TB accounts for the difficulty in its investigation; radiological imaging techniques and histopathology remain the gold standard (See Fig. 8.5) [23].

8.11   Brain TB and HANDS (Please Also See Chap. 9 for Further Details on TB Affecting the CNS)

The clinical presentation of TB and/or HIV infection is heterogeneous. Patients can present acutely with loss of consciousness, headaches, or with more chronic symptoms of cognitive deterioration. MRI is the mainstay diagnostic imaging investigation of intracranial space-occupying lesions (SOL); however this modality is not readily available in most developing countries. The brain is susceptible to

Fig. 8.5 Maximum intensity projection (MIP) images of an HIV-negative 33-year-old male who presented with chronic scrotal skin changes (i.e., skin thickening). Histopathology reported "granulomatous necrosis." He was placed on anti-TB therapy and steroids

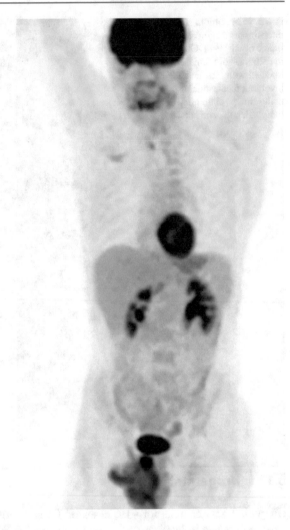

involvement with TB; in tuberculomas or HIV-associated neurocognitive disorders (HANDS), these conditions can be imaged medically in order to detect the clinical findings (See Fig. 8.6).

In a prospective study done by Gambhir and his colleagues to evaluate 10 patients with central nervous system (CNS) tuberculosis, it was concluded that FDG PET was complementary to MRI and detected more lesions extracranially [24].

PET imaging with ^{18}F-FDG PET can be used in the detection of SOL and in HANDS; however, it is not specific, and more specific tracers are being developed that would improve the diagnostic confidence in HIV and TB investigations [9, 18, 25–27].

Fig. 8.6 ^{18}F-FDG PET brain (axial) of a 41-year-old male, HIV-reactive with T-cell CD4 count >128 cell/mm^3, complaining of visual disturbances. Image findings were of multiple sites of TB tuberculomas. He was placed on an extended schedule of anti-TB treatment and demonstrated clinical improvement after 2 months

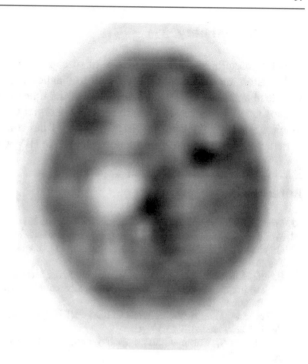

8.12   AIDS-Defining Illnesses

AIDS is the spectrum of HIV that is defined by the presence of one or more of several conditions associated with a reduced CD4 T-cell population and increased replication of the virus [18].

8.13 ^{18}F-FDG PET and HIV-Associated Cancers

- Kaposi's sarcoma demonstrates nonspecific accumulation of ^{18}F-FDG; additional research with newer tracers may yield more accurate results, averting the need for histopathology [28].
- The prevalence of invasive cervical carcinoma had been declining. PET imaging with FDG for locally advanced cervical carcinoma currently occurs routinely mainly due to the benefits of improved progression-free survival, disease-free survival, and overall survival; this work was described by Kidd et al. [29, 30].

8.14   In Summary

HIV-1 coinfection is the leading cause of susceptibility to TB; it alters the clinical presentation and makes it more difficult to diagnose. A careful history, results of viral load and CD4 count, and knowledge of the time of initiation of antiretroviral therapy are all necessary in order to correctly interpret an ^{18}F-FDG-PET/CT used to monitor treatment response in TB. ^{18}F-FDG PET has complementary clinical value in better understanding of the immune response in HIV–tuberculosis.

References

1. World Health Organization. Global tuberculosis report. 2018.
2. World Health Organization. End TB strategy. http://www.who.int/tb/strategy/end-tb/en/).
3. Gambhir S, Ravina M, Rangan K, et al. Imaging in extrapulmonary tuberculosis. Int J Infect Dis. 2017;56:237–47.
4. Esmail H, Riou C, Bruyn ED, Lai RP, Harley YXR, Meintjes G, Wilkinson KA, Wilkinson RJ. The immune response to Mycobacterium tuberculosis in HIV-1-coinfected persons. Annu Rev Immunol. 2018;36:603–38.
5. Sathekge M, Maes A, Van de Wiele C. FDG-PET imaging in HIV infection and tuberculosis. Semin Nucl Med. 2013;43:349–66.
6. Swanstrom R, Coffin J. HIV-1 pathogenesis. Cold Spring Harb Med Perspect Med. 2012;2:a007443.
7. Lackner A, Lederman M, Rodrigues B. HIV pathogenesis: the host. Cold Spring Harb Perspect Med. 2012;2:a007005.
8. https://wwwn.cdc.gov/hivrisk/what_is/stages_hiv_infection.html. Accessed 13 December 2018
9. Maartens G, Wilkinson RJ. Tuberculosis. Lancet. 2007;370(9604):2030–43. Epub 2007/08/28. S0140-6736(07)61262-8 [pii] pmid:17719083
10. Glaudemans W, Signore A. FDG-PET/CT in infections: the imaging method of choice? Eur J Nucl Med Mol Imaging. 2010;37:1986–91.
11. Keidar Z, Gurman-Balbir A, Gaitini D, et al. Fever of unknown origin: the role of FDG-PET/CT. J Nucl Med. 2008;49:1980–5.
12. Bleeker-Rovers CP, van der Meer JW, Oyen WJ. Fever of unknown origin. Semin Nucl Med. 2009;39:81–7.
13. Blocksman D, Knockaets D, Maes A, et al. Clinical value of FDG PET in patients with fever of unknown origin. Clin Infect Dis. 2001;32:191–6.
14. Subramanian S, Tawakol A, Burdo TH, et al. Arterial inflammation in patients with HIV. J Am Med Assoc. 2012;308:379–86.
15. Lee V, Wong J, Fan H, et al. Tuberculous pericarditis presenting as a massive pericardial effusion. BMJ Case Rep. 7:bcr0320125967.
16. Mayosi B, Burgess L, Doubel A. Tuberculous pericarditis. Circulation. 2005;112:3608–16.
17. Ntsheke M, Mayosi B. Tuberculous pericarditis with and without HIV. Heart Fail Rev. 2013;18:367–73.
18. https://www.ucsfhealth.org/conditions/aids/diagnosis.html. Accessed 12 December 2018.
19. Palestro C. Radionuclide imaging of musculoskeletal infection: a review. JNM. 2016;57(9):1406–12.
20. Leong AS-Y, Wannakrairot P, Leong TY-M. Apoptosis is a major cause of so-called "caseous necrosis" in mycobacterial granulomas in HIV-infected patients. J Clin Pathol. 2008;61(3):366–72.
21. Dureja S, Sen IB, Acharya S. Potential role of F18 FDG PET-CT as an imaging biomarker for the non-invasive evaluation in uncomplicated skeletal tuberculosis: a prospective clinical observation study. Eur Spine J. 2014;23:2449–54.

22. Lee G, Lee JH, Park SG. F-18 FDG PET/CT imaging of solitary genital tuberculosis mimicking recurrent lymphoma. Clin Nucl Med. 2011;36:315–6.
23. Kulchavenya E. Urogenital tuberculosis. Ther Adv Infect Dis. 2014;2:117–22.
24. Gambhir S, Kumar M, Ravina M, et al. Role of ^{18}F-FDG PET in demonstrating disease burden in patients tuberculous meningitis. J Neurol Sci. 2016;370:196–200.
25. Pelletier-Galarneau M, Martineau P, Zuckier L, et al. 18F-FDG-PET/CT imaging of thoracic and extrathoracic tuberculosis in children. Semin Nucl Med. 2013;43:349–66.
26. Ankrah A, Glaudemans A, Maes A, et al. Tuberculosis. Semin Nucl Med. 2017;48:108–30.
27. Sathekge M, Maes A, Kgomo M, et al. Impact of FDG PET on the management of TBC treatment. A pilot study. Nuklearmedizin. 2010;49:35–40.
28. Mankia SK, Miller RF, Edwards SG, et al. The response of HIV-associated lymphadenopathic kaposi sarcoma to highly active antiretroviral therapy evaluated by 18F-FDG PET/CT. Clin Nucl Med. 2012;37(7):692–3.
29. Sathekge M, Maes A, Van de Wiele C, et al. Effects of AIDS on women who have sex determined health issues. Semin Nucl Med. 2014;44:489–98.
30. Kidd E, Naqa I, Barry A, et al. FDG-PET-based prognostic nomograms for locally advanced cervical cancer. Gynecol Oncol. 2012;127:136–40.

Role of PET-CT in Central Nervous System Tuberculosis

9

Sanjay Gambhir, Kasturi Rangan, and Manish Ora

Contents

9.1   Introduction

About one third of the world's population is infected with tuberculous bacillus at this time frame, of which approximately 5–10% will manifest disease at some time during their life. India is front runner in incidence of tuberculosis (TB), carting a burden of 27% of the total world TB cases and harbouring approximately 10.4 million cases [1]. It is estimated that 4.5 lakh people die every year with TB. In 2014, the World Health Assembly pledged a strategy to end tuberculosis, with a goal of achieving reduction of incidence of TB globally by less than 50% and reducing mortality by less than 75% by 2025 and an overall 2035 target of 90% reduction in incidence and 95% reduction in mortality [2].

Neurotuberculosis constitutes 1% of all tuberculosis and 10–15% of the extra-pulmonary tuberculosis cases, mostly seen among children (~40%) [3]. Central nervous system (CNS) tuberculosis is associated with 1.5–3.2% of all tuberculosis-related deaths [4]. Tubercular bacilli start granulomatous inflammation in different brain

S. Gambhir (✉) · K. Rangan · M. Ora
Department of Nuclear Medicine, S.G.P.G.I.M.S, Lucknow, India

© Springer Nature Switzerland AG 2020
D. Sobic Saranovic et al. (eds.), *PET/CT in Tuberculosis*, Clinicians' Guides to Radionuclide Hybrid Imaging, https://doi.org/10.1007/978-3-030-47009-8_9

tissues like meninges, brain parenchyma, spinal cord and skull bones. The CNS manifestations are in varied forms, such as tubercular meningitis (TBM), cerebritis, tuberculoma, and abscess. Spinal cord involvement is less common and seen as arachnoiditis and/or intramedullary tuberculoma [5].

Early diagnosis and treatment of CNS tuberculosis are very important to reduce the morbidity and mortality. Non-invasive imaging modalities such as computed tomography (CT) and magnetic resonance imaging (MRI) are used commonly for the diagnosis of CNS TB [5]. CT and MRI provide excellent structural resolution of the inflammatory and infective pathologies. However, these anatomical imaging modalities are of limited value in detecting early metabolic changes that occur in inflammatory disorders. Benign diseases such as infection, inflammation, and chronic granulomatous conditions appear to have increased glycolysis and therefore are seen on 18F-fluorodeoxyglucose (18F-FDG) positron emission tomography (PET) [6]. The role of FDG in infectious and inflammatory diseases is evolving, and there are very few studies on the role of 18F-FDG PET/CT in TBM [7]. This article reviews the various forms of CNS tuberculosis, including its complications and imaging features on PET/CT concentrating on 18F-FDG PET/CT.

9.2   Pathophysiology

TBM—(Fig. 9.1) It presents as primary infection in childhood and a post-primary infection in adulthood [5]. It spread hematogenously from distant active sites such as the lung, bone, lymph nodes and gastrointestinal or genitourinary tract. Infection typically begins in a subpial or subependymal region called the Rich focus [8]. Initially, a non-specific inflammatory reaction, tuberculous cerebritis, starts. After sensitisation, inflammatory response results in a granuloma which erodes into the subarachnoid space and cerebrospinal fluid (CSF), causing basal leptomeningitis. Subsequently, this leads to communicating hydrocephalus and occasionally obstructive hydrocephalus by obstruction of the foramina of Luschka and Magendie. Vasculitis may occur with involvement of lenticulostriate and thalamoperforating arteries. Reactive subendothelial cellular proliferation may lead to vascular obstruction and cause small infarcts in the deep grey matter nuclei and deep white matter [9]. Extra-pulmonary TB occurs in up to 50% of these patients, which provide helpful clue to diagnosis [10].

Tuberculoma—It is an initial lesion consisting of a central area of incipient or frank necrosis surrounded by inflammatory cells, lymphocytes, epithelioid cells and Langhans giant cells, with an encircling rich vascular zone. A few bacilli may be present in the centre. The caseation then usually liquefies from the centre. The capsule consists of granulation tissue and compressed glial tissue [5]. FDG PET-CT shows a "doughnut" appearance with intense tracer uptake at the periphery and low central uptake [11].

TB infection in the spine—It may involve any compartment in the spinal region, i.e. vertebrae, intervertebral disk, spinal cord and meninges. Meningeal involvement leads to spinal meningitis and spinal arachnoiditis. The pathophysiology of spinal meningitis is the same as described earlier in TBM [12].

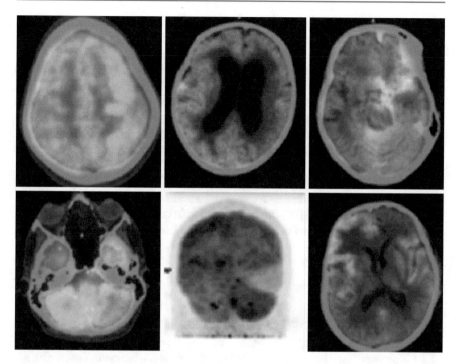

Fig. 9.1 Various types of CNS tubercular lesions as seen in FDG PET-CT, clockwise from upper left corner: tuberculoma, hydrocephalus, basal exudates, leptomeningeal enhancement, vascular infarct, cerebellar lesions

9.3 Clinical Features

Children and older people are susceptible to TBM. TBM is seen commonly in immune-compromised patients (HIV/AIDS, diabetes, patients taking immune-suppressive medication such as steroids or cytotoxic drugs). Initial presentation is nausea, vomiting, headache, neck stiffness and photophobia [13]. Cranial nerve palsies, especially of third, fourth and sixth, may also be seen. Tuberculomas manifest like space-occupying lesion, and the patients present with features of increased intracranial pressure, focal or generalised seizures and focal neurologic deficit.

9.3.1 Limitations and Challenges of TB Diagnostics

Microbiological demonstration of tuberculosis remains difficult due to difficult sampling, low yield and long culture time (6–8 weeks). Thus the index of suspicion is mostly indirect, that is, concomitant tubercular involvement elsewhere, malaise, low-grade fever, weight loss, positive tuberculin test, raised ESR and history of contact [14]. CSF analysis in TBM may show a lymphocytic pleocytosis, increased protein and decreased glucose level [15]. CSF culture for acid-fast bacilli and CSF polymerase chain reaction (PCR) examination are confirmatory tests for the diagnosis of TBM [15, 16]. Meticulous microscopy of large CSF volumes improves sensitivity, but it rarely exceeds 60% [16]. Nucleic acid amplification technique (NAAT) is only 56% sensitive (95% CI 46–66) and 98% specific. It can confirm a diagnosis of TM but cannot rule it out [17]. The Xpert MTB/RIF assay uses real-time PCR and has become cornerstone of commercial molecular diagnosis. It may confirm *M. tuberculosis* in CSF and its susceptibility to rifampicin within 2 h, although its value in the diagnosis of tuberculous meningitis remains uncertain. Xpert MTB/RIF shows ~80% sensitivity compared with culture for the diagnosis of extra-pulmonary tuberculosis [18].

Anti-tuberculous therapy is recommended for 9 to 12 months. Adjunctive corticosteroid therapy for the initial 6–8 weeks is associated with reduced mortality and fewer neurologic sequelae [19]. Mortality is high in patients younger than 5 years, those older than 50 years and those in whom illness has been present for longer than 2 months [20].

9.3.2 Imaging

Imaging protocol for 18F FDG PET-CT—In our institute, whole-body PET-CT image acquisition with separate brain protocol is performed with an integrated PET-CT system (True Point PET-CT System, Biograph 64, Siemens, Germany). All the patients must have blood glucose less than 150 mg/dl and should be fasting for 6 h before the scan. Patients are made to rest in a dim lit room for 30 min, and then they are given intravenous injection of 10 mCi (370 MBq) followed by resting period for 60 more minutes. Whole-body PET/CT scanning with arms up position is acquired with 64-slice spiral MDCT, using acquisition parameters of 120 keV and tube current of 200 mA, with a pitch ratio of 0.8 and slice thickness of 0.5 mm, followed by PET acquisition at the identical axial field of view (FOV). A separate brain acquisition is done using PET reconstruction of 400 $*$ 400, OSEM 3D 2i24S, XYZ Gauss 2.00. PET image data sets are reconstructed iteratively with segmented correction for attenuation, scatter and decay with the use of the CT data. The images are reconstructed in trans-axial, sagittal and coronal slices [21].

9.3.3 Assessment of Disease

9.3.3.1 Cranial Tuberculosis

TBM
Meninges are involved either by hematogenous seeding or by local spread from adjoining infected areas. In the early stages, conventional non-contrast MR imaging studies usually show little or no evidence of any meningeal abnormality. However FDG PET-CT has very high sensitivity to detect changes in early stages of disease. As the disease progresses, FDG uptake with abnormal meningeal enhancement is

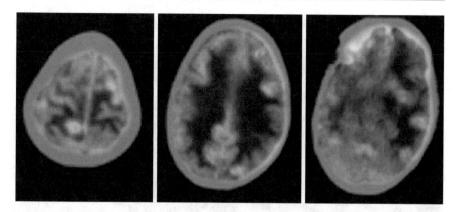

Fig. 9.2 A 36-year-old male presented with seizures and headache for 2 weeks. CSF examination (lymphocytosis with increased proteins and decreased glucose) and MRI (multiple tuberculomas with few subcortical areas of diffusion restrictions and vasogenic oedema) were done. FDG PET-CT revealed well-defined ring-enhancing tuberculoma (upper left), leptomeningeal enhancements with oedema (middle) and multiple patchy nodular lesions in left frontal and parietal regions

commonly seen in interpeduncular fossa, pontine cistern, perimesencephalic cistern, suprasellar cistern, and Sylvian fissures, with occasional involvement of sulci over the convexities [21–23] (Fig. 9.2).

Hydrocephalus (Fig. 9.1)
It may develop as a result of blockage of the basal cisterns by the inflammatory exudates (communicating type) (see Fig. 9.1), due to mass effect of a focal parenchymal lesion or entrapment of the ventricle by granulomatous ependymitis. Atrophy of brain parenchyma is a late sequela of chronic hydrocephalus. The choroid plexus may serve as an entry point for the pathogens into the CNS. Its involvement, choroid plexitis, presents as prominent contrast enhancement of the choroid plexus and is usually associated with ependymitis, ventriculitis and meningitis [5].

Vasculitis
Vasculitis is another common complication of TBM involving small- and medium-sized vessels and causing ischemic cerebral infarction [24]. Most of the infarcts are in the region of basal ganglia and internal capsule due to involvement of the lenticulostriate arteries; however, involvement of the artery such as the middle cerebral artery may also be encountered (Fig. 9.3) [25]. Vascular complications are usually seen following initiation of specific therapy, possibly due to the healing and fibrosis of meninges resulting in the occlusion of embedded vasculature.

Cranial Nerve Neuropathy
It is seen in 17.4–40% of patients by vascular compromise resulting in ischemia of the nerve or by entrapment of the nerves by the exudate [26]. Evaluation of nerves is better appreciated in MRI due to its superior spatial and contrast resolution.

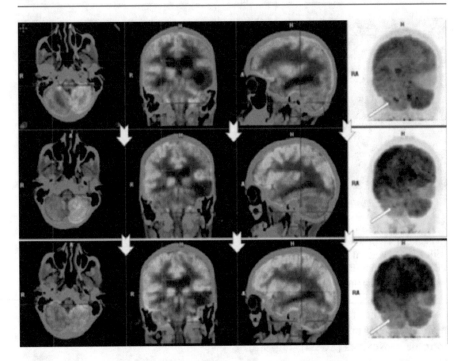

Fig. 9.3 Three follow-up FDG PET-CT scans showing insult to left MCA territory with crossed cerebellar diaschisis and cerebellar tuberculoma (upper row). No significant improvement was noted in the infarcted site; however, there was improvement in the symptoms and grade normalization of the crossed cerebellar diaschisis

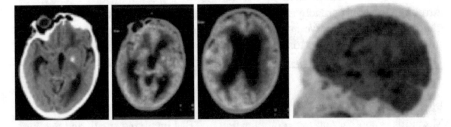

Fig. 9.4 It shows a calcified focus with no FDG avidity and is associated with multiple active tuberculomas and hydrocephalus

Intracranial Tuberculoma (Fig. 9.4)

It is a space-occupying mass of granulomatous tissue that is encountered more frequently in developing countries [27]. Early recognition and treatment of this condition on imaging play an important role in patient management. Intracranial tuberculomas may be solitary or multiple and are of variable size [28]. These tuberculomas are found across all age groups; however, a predilection for children has been reported. The common sites include cerebral hemispheres, basal ganglia, cerebellum and brainstem. Rarely, ventricular system and meninges are also involved

[29]. In acute phase this tuberculoma shows FDG avidly, and in the later phases, it shows doughnut sign. In chronic state only a calcified nodule is seen with no metabolic activity.

Tuberculous Brain Abscess

It constitutes approximately 4–7% of the total CNS TB in developing countries. These abscesses are diagnosed from macroscopic evidence of abscess formation along with histologic demonstration of vascular granulation tissue in the wall containing both acute and chronic inflammatory cells and isolation of *M. tuberculosis* [30]. Possibility of a tuberculous brain abscess should be considered when FDG accumulates at the periphery of a ring-enhancing lesion with low uptake in the centre in a chronically ill or immunocompromised patient [31].

9.3.3.2 Spinal Tuberculosis (Fig. 9.5)

Intraspinal TB

In arachnoiditis, imaging features include CSF loculation and obliteration of the spinal subarachnoid space with loss of outline of the spinal cord and clumping of the nerve roots. Contrast MR studies may show nodular, thick, linear dural enhancement, often completely filling the subarachnoid space on post-contrast [32]. In chronic stages of the disease, signs of arachnoiditis are noted with no significant enhancement. The spinal cord may be involved secondarily and show infarction, syringomyelia, myelitis and tuberculoma formation [33]. FDG avidity may be seen in all the pathologies like arachnoiditis, spinal tuberculoma, myelitis and infarction.

Myelitis (Fig. 9.5)

Tuberculous myelitis is usually associated with tubercular meningitis, involvement of brain parenchyma or tuberculous arachnoiditis. Intramedullary tuberculomas are

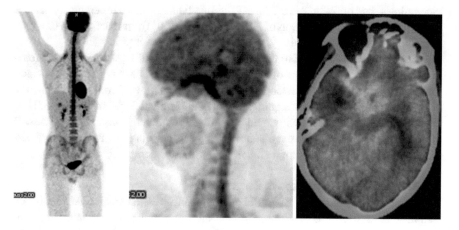

Fig. 9.5 FDG PET-CT showing diffuse uptake along the spinal cord, with multiple tuberculomas and basal exudate

uncommon and have similar imaging features to brain tuberculomas [34]. Earlier phases of the reactive process show high FDG avidity.

Dural and Subdural Disorders

Tuberculous pus formation may occur between the dura and leptomeninges, and it appears as a loculation. Epidural tuberculous abscesses may be seen in isolation or in association with arachnoiditis, myelitis, spondylitis and intramedullary and dural tuberculomas [34].

Tuberculous Spondylitis

Tuberculous spondylitis is a frequent-occurrence in developing countries and is an important cause of spine-related morbidity. Early diagnosis and prompt treatment are required to avoid permanent deformity. It involves vertebral bodies and regional structure such as posterior osseous elements, epidural space, paraspinal soft tissue and intervertebral disc. It most commonly involves dorsal and lumbar spine, especially the thoracolumbar junction. Usually more than one vertebral body is affected, but solitary vertebral lesions can also occur. Marrow abnormalities occur before any bony destruction. As the disease progresses, discovertebral involvement may be visible. Features such as vertebral intraosseous abscesses, paraspinal abscesses, discitis, skip lesions, and spinal canal encroachment may be seen. Reduction in disk height and morphologic alteration of the paraspinal soft tissue are late occurrences. Demonstration of bone fragments in the intraspinal and/or extraspinal soft tissue is considered characteristic of tuberculous spondylitis. This is caused by the lack of proteolytic enzymes that lyse the bone in the tuberculous inflammatory exudate. These fragments are best shown on PET-CT [35] (Fig. 9.6).

9.3.3.3 Tuberculosis in HIV/AIDS

Tuberculosis has seen a resurgence in the past two decades because of the increasing numbers of patients with AIDS. A total of 5–9% of patients with AIDS develop tuberculosis, and of these, 2–18% have CNS involvement. CNS tuberculosis may be the initial clinical manifestation of AIDS and may result from reactivation of a previous infection or from a primary, newly acquired infection [36].

The value of PET applied to the metabolic evaluation of HIV and TB is increasingly recognised. Knowledge of varied spectrum of AIDS-defining illnesses and immunovirological status is essential for interpreting FDG-PET imaging. FDG-PET holds great potential to play a significant role in the clinical decision-making of HIV patients presenting with AIDS-related opportunistic infections and malignancies. It provides appropriate differential diagnoses, suggests correlation with laboratory and microbiological assays or biopsy, and reliably assesses therapeutic response.

9.3.3.4 Documenting Disease Burden

Being a whole-body study, FDG PET/CT not only demonstrates distribution of lesion; it guides for site of biopsy or aspiration and assists in surgical planning. Many patients who presented with CNS TB show extracranial lesions which can provide a less invasive site for biopsy.

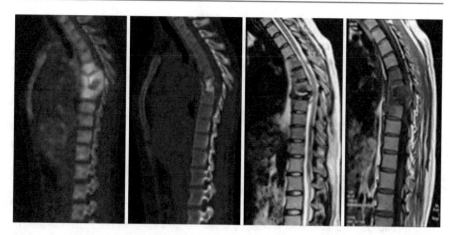

Fig. 9.6 Sagittal FDG PET-CT of Pott's spine showing involvement of mid-dorsal vertebrae and its correlation with MRI (T2 and T1 images) revealing multi-level partial compression fracture of the vertebrae and significant metabolic activity

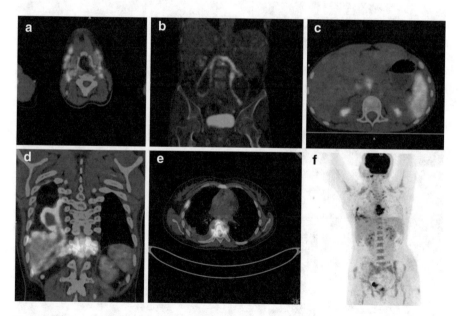

Fig. 9.7 Demonstrating various tubercular lesions in the body such as (**a**) tubercular lymphade-nopathy, (**b**) psoas abscess, (**c**) retroperitoneal lymphadenopathy with splenic involvement, (**d**) perihepatic abscess, (**e**) rib lesion, (**f**) bone marrow activation

The extent and metabolic activity of disease on the baseline FDG PET-CT demonstrate disease burden and prognosis in individual patient. Higher uptake in the brain tuberculomas with nerve and basal exudation may have poor prognosis. Follow-up of these patients with PET-CT scan is recommended as they may have varied course of treatment response to standard medications. Few of them can

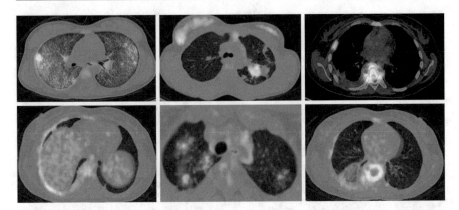

Fig. 9.8 Patterns of extra-cranial pulmonary lesions (clockwise from the upper left corner), military tubercle, consolidation, pleural effusion, fibro-consolidatory changes, reticulonodular opacities (tree in bud appearance), pleural thickening

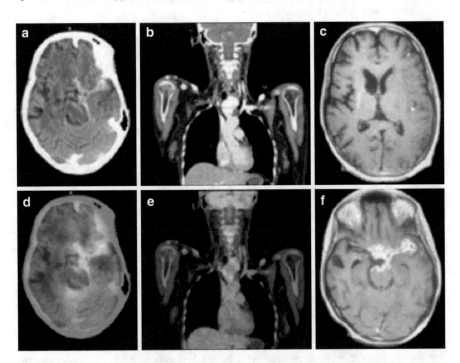

Fig. 9.9 Enhancing metabolically active tubercular basal exudate, with carotid artery aneurysm

show resistance to one or more drugs, which may be seen on interim FDG PET-CT scans. Alterations in the treatment may be warranted to avoid futile treatment.

The penultimate question which is always bombarding the physician is the right time to stop anti-tubercular medications in these patients. This could be accessed with the help of FDG PET-CT. Hence it may guide in establishing a therapeutic end point (Figs. 9.7–9.9).

9.3.3.5 Dual Time Point Imaging

Studies have documented the value of additional delayed images at 90–120 min after injection, in differentiating benign from malignant lesions. On delayed images, inflammatory lesions show FDG washout, whereas malignant lesions usually exhibit accumulation of tracer. In our experience majority of the tuberculous lesions showed no reduction; only few of them showed mild reduction (up to 20%) (Fig. 9.10).

9.3.3.6 Assessment of Therapeutic Response

Abnormalities detected on baseline MRI and CT may take months to years to normalise. Metabolic activity of the lesion may play an important role in determining activity in a residual lesion and may guide an appropriate time to stop medication. Serial imaging in responding patients shows a decrease in lesion size and significant decrease in metabolic activity after 3–4 months and its disappearance by 1 year. Rarely, a progression of intracranial tuberculomas or development of new lesions during the treatment of CNS tuberculosis has also been recognised. Calcification of the meninges and parenchymal tuberculoma are seen as sequelae of TBM [37] (Figs. 9.11 and 9.12).

9.3.3.7 Drawbacks of FDG PET-CT

1. Infection, inflammation and granulomatous lesion may have FDG uptake due to increased glucose metabolism by macrophages and inflammatory cells; hence, it has low specificity.
2. Corticosteroid may result in membrane stabilization, reduced inflammation and increased blood sugar level, which may decrease or absent FDG uptake resulting in false-negative result. A lesion with low uptake adjacent to another highly active lesion may show reduced FDG uptake.
3. Seizure produced generalised increased metabolic activity and small lesion may be hindered, or focal seizure may reveal focal FDG uptake without structural lesion.
4. Due to lower spatial resolution of PET, sub-centimetre lesion may show decreased or absent metabolic activity.
5. Brain parenchyma shows physiological uptake which may show no differential uptake in the lesion due to low contrast resolution.

9.3.3.8 Quantitative Analysis

The relevance of loss of cerebral function after infective sequelae is not well understood in patients with TBM. Clinical and neurophysiological studies provide adequate evidence supporting reorganisation of the function centres in brain post trauma/infection. However this reorganisation is not well studied in terms of brain metabolism. Future studies that utilise neurological quantification algorithms to elicit the functional changes in brain after infective sequelae are warranted (Fig. 9.13).

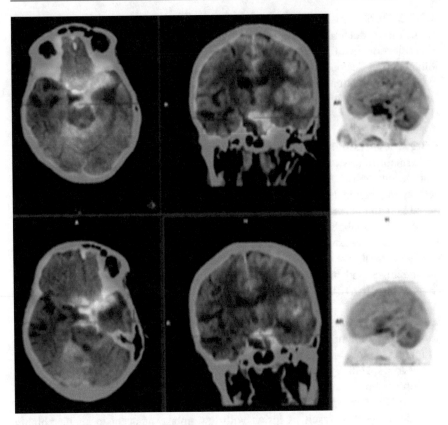

Fig. 9.10 Dual point imaging of a patient at 60 and 120 min (upper and lower rows). Basal exudates show ~20% reduction in the metabolism, with stable contrast retention

9.3.3.9 Tuberculosis Specific Imaging and Its Role in Pharmacology and Drug Development Research

Deep seated infections and CNS tubercular infections are always a diagnostic challege, as tissue biopsies are difficult. Obtaining samples is not only time-consuming but also dangerous and expensive. The results can take several days and may not always provide reliable holistic information about TB and disease burden. Also, traditional methos are inadequate to answer some important questions regarding disease distribution in the whole body, interaction of the medication with the targets and disease modification during the course of treatment [38]. PET imaging provides a true solution for molecular imaging as most small molecules can be efficiently labelled with 11C or with 18F at >37 GBq/μmol (1 Ci/μmol), and they can be detected with PET in the nanomolar to picomolar concentration range [39].

PET imaging may be done even when total amount of a radiotracer administered is extremely low (microdosing, typically <1 μg for humans). It is very valuable for evaluating tissue exposure in the early phase of drug development when the full-range toxicology is not yet available [40]. PET imaging may be used for quantitative

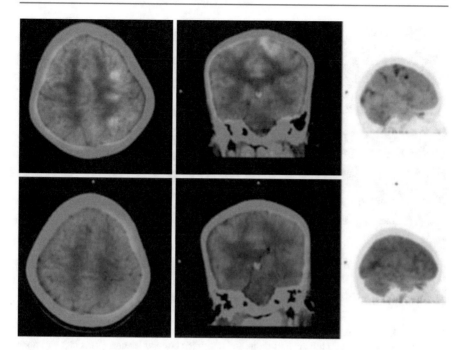

Fig. 9.11 Baseline and follow-up at 12 months (upper and lower rows) showing complete metabolic response of the tubercular lesions

information of drug pharmacokinetic (PK) and distribution in various tissues including brain; confirming drug binding with targets and elucidating the relationship between occupancy and target expression/function in vivo; assessing drug passage across the blood-brain barrier and ensuring sufficient exposure to the brain for central nervous system drugs; and dissecting the modifying effects of drugs on diseases [41].

The current treatment regime for drug-sensitive TB involves the use of rifampicin (RIF), INH, pyrazinamide (PZA) and ethambutol or streptomycin. This regime is primarily based on pharmacokinetic studies in serum and on efficacy of treatment. The efficacy of each drug for different types of TB such as brain TB and the drug distribution in other organs are not well understood. A major advantage of the technique is measure in situ PK in real-time, and simultaneously in multiple organ system or compartments with relatively unaltered physiology. As plasma levels may not reflect tissue PK, nuclear imaging with radiolabelled drugs could provide detailed preclinical data for appropriate dosing of new TB drugs, both to ensure sufficient drug in target tissue and to evaluate for its presence in sites of potential toxicity [42].

Liu et al. labelled INH, RIF and PZA with 11C and used PET to investigate their PK and biodistribution in baboons. They found that the organ distribution and BBB penetration of each drug differed greatly. The ability of [11C]INH to penetrate the BBB was lower than that of PZA but higher than that of RIF (PZA > INH > RIF).

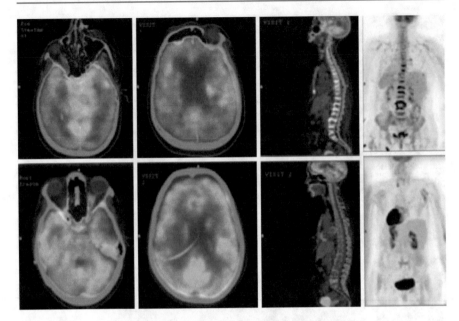

Fig. 9.12 Baseline and follow-up at 12 months (upper and lower rows) showing complete metabolic response of the brain tubercular lesions and multiple vertebral lesions. (VP shunt was done for decompression)

The INH concentrations in the lungs and brain were ten times higher than the INH minimum inhibitory concentration (MIC) value against TB, supporting the use of INH for treating TB infections in the lungs and brain [43].

First-in-human 11C-rifampin PET imaging performed in a patient with TBM confirmed these findings. Author demonstrated that rifampin penetration into infected brain lesions is limited, is heterogeneous and decreases rapidly as early as 2 weeks into treatment. Moreover, rifampin concentrations in the cerebrospinal fluid did not correlate well with those in the brain lesions. PK modelling predicted that rifampin doses (≥30 mg/kg) are required to achieve adequate intralesional concentrations in young children with TBM. These data demonstrate the proof of concept of PET as a clinically unparalleled tool to non-invasively measure intralesional antimicrobial distribution in infected tissues [44].

9.4   Conclusion

Tuberculosis is omnipresent and may involve virtually every organ system. Whole-body PET-CT scan in a single study provides all relevant anatomical and functional information about the tuberculosis burden and provides the distribution, extent, biopsy site and even prognosticate disease. Hence it is a single stop shop modality for this magnanimous disease. It can also help in making decision for appropriate antibiotic therapy, treatment follow up and establishing therapeutic end points. This is important because current standand investigations have difficulty in prospectively

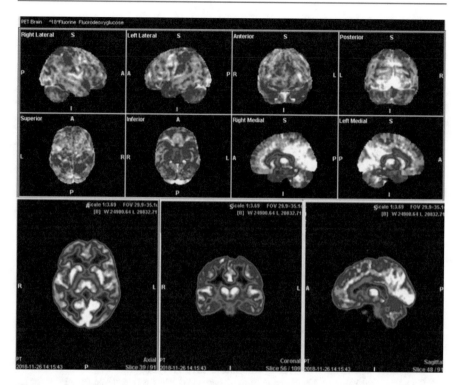

Fig. 9.13 Global view of the quantitative analysis of the patient with CNS tuberculosis, showing multiple areas of hypometabolism around the tuberculomas indicating vasogenic oedema

predicting those patients who may relapse and require additional months of treatment.

Development of tuberculosis specific radioligands and improved image analysis have potential to give real-time insight of complex microbiological, immunological and physiological states of the disease in living hosts and effect of treatment on them. In coming years PET-CT will aid in understanding TB, providing personalised clinical management and can accelerate the development of new therapeutics with lesser side effects.

Acknowledgement We appreciate IAEA for supporting our dedicated work on tuberculosis.

Use of 18F-FDG PET/CT for Imaging TB Patients and Related Conditions (HIV/AIDS, Tuberculosis): Focus on Drug Resistant Extrapulmonary Tuberculosis. IAEA, CRP E15021.

References

1. WHO 2018/2019 tuberculosis global facts. https://www.who.int/features/factfiles/tuberculosis/en/. Accessed Feb 2019.
2. Verguet S, Riumallo-Herl C, Gomez GB, et al. Catastrophic costs potentially averted by tuberculosis control in India and South Africa: a modelling study. Lancet Glob Health. 2017;5(11):e1123–32.

3. Garg RK. Classic diseases revisited: tuberculosis of the central nervous system. Postgrad Med J. 1999;75:133–40.
4. Rock RB, Olin M, Baker CA, et al. Central nervous system tuberculosis: pathogenesis and clinical aspects. Clin Microbiol Rev. 2008;21:243–61.
5. Rakesh KG, Sunil K. Central nervous system tuberculosis. Neuroimaging Clin N Am. 2011;21:795–814.
6. Yuichi I, Yasuo K, Sasaki M, et al. FDG-PET in infectious lesions: the detection and assessment of lesion activity. Ann Nucl Med. 1996;10:185–91.
7. Omri HE, Hascsi Z, Taha R, et al. Tubercular meningitis and lymphadenitis mimicking a relapse of Burkitt's lymphoma on ^{18}F-FDG-PET/CT: a case report. Case Rep Oncol. 2015;8(2):226–32.
8. Garcia-Monco JC. Central nervous system tuberculosis. Neurol Clin. 1999;17:737–59.
9. Dastur DK, Manghani DK, Udani PM. Pathology and pathogenic mechanisms in neurotuberculosis. Radiol Clin N Am. 1995;33:733–52.
10. Bernaerts A, Vanhoenacker FM, Parizel PM, et al. Tuberculosis of the central nervous system: overview of neuroradiological findings. Eur Radiol. 2003;13:1876–90.
11. Harkirat S, Anana SS, et al. Pictorial essay: PET/CT in tuberculosis. Indian J Radiol Imaging. 2008;18(2):141–7.
12. Brooks WD, Fletcher AP, Wilson RR. Spinal cord complications of tuberculous meningitis; a clinical and pathological study. Q J Med. 1954;23:275–90.
13. Leonard JM, Des Prez RM. Tuberculous meningitis. Infect Dis Clin N Am. 1990;4:769–87.
14. Dott NM, Levine E. Intracranial tuberculoma. Edinb Med J. 1939;46:36–41.
15. Kennedy DH, Fallon RJ. Tuberculous meningitis. JAMA. 1979;241:264–8.
16. Zuger A, Lowy FD. Tuberculosis. In: Scheld WM, Whitley RJ, Durack DT, editors. Infection of the central nervous system. 2nd ed. Philadelphia, PA: Lippincott-Raven; 1997. p. 417–43.
17. Gupta R, Talwar P, et al. Diagnostic accuracy of nucleic acid amplification based assays for tuberculous meningitis: a meta-analysis. J Infect. 2018;77(4):302–13.
18. Kim MJ, Nam YS, et al. Comparison of the Xpert MTB/RIF assay and real-time PCR for the detection of Mycobacterium tuberculosis. Ann Clin Lab Sci. 2015;45(3):327–32.
19. Sophie J, Hannah R, et al. Six months therapy for tuberculous meningitis. Cochrane Database Syst Rev. 2016;9:1–112.
20. Peter JD, Courtney MY, et al. The global burden of tuberculosis mortality in children: a mathematical modelling study. Lancet Glob Health. 2017;5(9):e898–906.
21. Gambhir S, Kumar M, et al. Role of F-18 FDG PET in demonstrating disease burden in patients with tuberculous meningitis. J Neurol Sci. 2016;370:196–200.
22. Kioumehr F, Dadsetan MR, Rooholamini AA. Central nervous system tuberculosis: MRI. Neuroradiology. 1994;36:93–6.
23. Whiteman M, Espinoza L, Post MJD, et al. Central nervous system tuberculosis in HIV-infected patients: clinical and radiographic findings. AJNR Am J Neuroradiol. 1995;16:1319–27.
24. Tandon PN, Bhatia R, Bhargava S. Tuberculous meningitis. In: Vinken PJ, Bruyn GW, Klawans HZ, editors. Handbook of clinical neurology, vol. 8. Amsterdam: Elsevier; 1988. p. 196–226.
25. Shukla R, Abbas A, Kumar P, et al. Evaluation of cerebral infarction in tuberculous meningitis by diffusion weighted imaging. J Infect. 2008;57:298–306.
26. Gupta RK. Tuberculosis and other non-tuberculous bacterial granulomatous infections. In: Gupta RK, Lufkin RB, editors. MR imaging and spectroscopy of central nervous system infection. New York: Kluwer Academic/Plenum Publishers; 2001. p. 95–145.
27. Tandon PN, Pathak SN. Tuberculosis of the central nervous system. In: Spillane JD, editor. Tropical neurology. New York: Oxford University Press; 1973. p. 37–62.
28. Gupta RK, Jena A, Sharma A, et al. MR imaging of intracranial tuberculomas. J Comput Assist Tomogr. 1988;12:280–5.
29. Whelan MA, Steven J. Intracranial tuberculoma. Radiology. 1981;138:75–81.
30. Whitener DR. Tuberculous brain abscess. Report of a case and review of the literature. Arch Neurol. 1978;35:148–55.

31. Kang K, Lim I, Roh JK. Positron emission tomographic findings in a tuberculous abscess. Ann Nucl Med. 2007;21:303–6.
32. Kumar A, Montanera W, Willinsky R, et al. MR features of tuberculous arachnoiditis. J Comput Assist Tomogr. 1993;17:127–30.
33. Gupta RK, Gupta S, Kumar S, et al. MRI in intraspinal tuberculosis. Neuroradiology. 1994;36:39–43.
34. Jena A, Banerji AK, Tripathi RP, et al. Demonstration of intramedullary tuberculomas by magnetic resonance imaging: a report of two cases. Br J Radiol. 1991;64:555–7.
35. Gupta RK, Agarwal P, Rastogi H, et al. Problems in differentiating spinal tuberculosis from neoplasm on MRI. Neuroradiology. 1996;38:S97–104.
36. Villoria MF, de la Torre J, Fortea F, et al. Intracranial tuberculosis in AIDS: CT and MRI findings. Neuroradiology. 1992;34:11–4.
37. Ku BD, Yoo SD. Extensive meningeal and parenchymal calcified tuberculoma as long-term residual sequelae of tuberculous meningitis. Neurol India. 2009;57:521–2.
38. Fox GB, Chin CL, Luo F, Day M, Cox BF. Translational neuroimaging of the CNS: novel pathways to drug development. Mol Interv. 2009;9(6):302–13.
39. Lee CM, Farde L. Using positron emission tomography to facilitate CNS drug development. Trends Pharmacol Sci. 2006;27(6):310–6.
40. Bauer M, Wagner CC, Langer O. Microdosing studies in humans: the role of positron emission tomography. Drugs R D. 2008;9(2):73–81.
41. Hammond LA, Denis L, Salman U, Jerabek P, Thomas CR Jr, Kuhn JG. Positron emission tomography (PET): expanding the horizons of oncology drug development. Investig New Drugs. 2003;21(3):309–40.
42. Matthews PM, Rabiner EA, Passchier J, Gunn RN. Positron emission tomography molecular imaging for drug development. Br J Clin Pharmacol. 2012;73:175–86.
43. Liu L, Xu Y, Shea C, Fowler JS, Hooker JM, Tonge PJ. Radiosynthesis and bioimaging of the tuberculosis chemotherapeutics isoniazid, rifampicin and pyrazinamide in baboons. J Med Chem. 2010;53(7):2882–91.
44. Tucker EW, Guglieri-lopez B, Ordonez AA, et al. Noninvasive C-rifampin positron emission tomography reveals drug biodistribution in tuberculous meningitis. Sci Transl Med. 2018;10(470):eaau0965.

FDG PET/CT in TB: Mimics, Pitfalls, and Limitations

10

Dragana Sobic Saranovic and Milica Stojiljkovic

Contents

Tuberculosis (TB) is known to be a great mimicker as it can masquerade as various number of inflammatory or malignant disorders. One of the main drawbacks of positron emission tomography/computed tomography with 18F-fluorodeoxyglucose (FDG PET/CT) is its lack of specificity in order to distinguish between different inflammations and/or malignancies (Fig. 10.1). When interpreting FDG PET/CT findings, it is important to consider that cancer patients are susceptible to develop active TB, with substantive increase of short-term risk among patients with cancers of aerodigestive tract and hematological cancers, but also markedly elevated risk in patients with tobacco-related cancers. In addition, cytostatics and radiotherapy further increase TB risk in oncological patients. TB occurrence in cancer patients is more than four times greater than in general population within the first year following diagnosis, with the incidence of TB in hematopoietic stem cell transplant recipients up to 16% [1, 2]. In patients with malignant hemopathy, tuberculin skin test is usually negative due to the defect in the immunity related to the disease itself and therapy [3], and radiological abnormalities may be minimal or atypical in patients

D. Sobic Saranovic (✉)
Faculty of Medicine, University of Belgrade, Belgrade, Serbia

Center for Nuclear Medicine, Clinical Center of Serbia, Belgrade, Serbia

M. Stojiljkovic
Center for Nuclear Medicine, Clinical Center of Serbia, Belgrade, Serbia

© Springer Nature Switzerland AG 2020
D. Sobic Saranovic et al. (eds.), *PET/CT in Tuberculosis*, Clinicians' Guides to Radionuclide Hybrid Imaging, https://doi.org/10.1007/978-3-030-47009-8_10

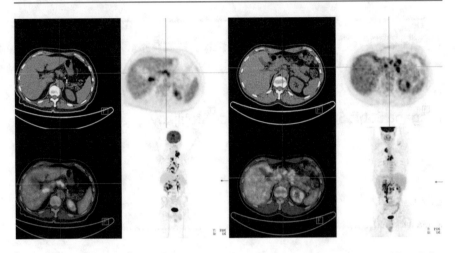

Fig. 10.1 Patient on the left presenting with tuberculous lymphadenitis on both sides of diaphragm; patient on the right showing metastatic lymph nodes in neck, mediastinum, and abdomen, due to colorectal carcinoma

with myelosuppression, with frequent extrapulmonary disease, so correct diagnosis often poses a challenge. Conversely, prolonged pulmonary inflammation in TB patients may cause tissue damage and genomic alterations, and repair of the damage can lead to pulmonary fibrosis and scarring, all of which being linked to increased lung cancer risk. Tuberculosis is associated with a twofold elevation in lung cancer risk, with greatest risk up to even fivefold elevation seen in the first 2 years after diagnosis of TB, but it remains elevated also at longer time periods [4]. The highest probability of detecting coexistent malignant disease in patients with granulomatous inflammations exists in patients over 60 years suffering from tuberculosis, where an important feature for identification of malignancy on FDG PET/CT, especially in the assessment of intrathoracic findings, turns out to be the CT pattern, with quantitative evaluation of metabolic activity, in contrast, having little clinical value [5]. That somewhat agrees with the reports of FDG PET/CT having higher degree of detection of metabolically active lesions in lung cancer patients compared to only morphological lesions seen on CT, since some of these foci could represent TB or other inflammatory processes [6]. There are numerous reports of active tuberculosis found on FDG PET/CT concomitantly with or following treatment of malignant disease, where sites of high metabolic activity could have and often were initially mistakenly proclaimed to be active malignancy, including patients with malignant melanoma and squamous cellular skin cancer; lung cancer; digestive system malignancies; kidney, prostate, breast, and cervical carcinomas; and various types of lymphomas, with SUVmax values detected in TB sites comparable to those in malignant lesions in the same patients [7–23].

PET was found to have high false-positive rate when evaluating solitary pulmonary nodules (SPN) in TB endemic areas, and combination of PET and CT (PET/CT) was suggested for improvement of the diagnostic accuracy in the differentiation of SPN [24]. Significant overlap can be seen in the degree of FDG uptake of malignant and tuberculous nodules without significant difference between their maximum standardized uptake (SUVmax) values, with highest recorded SUVmax of pulmonary TB lesions up to 22.5 [25, 26]. When the SUVmax of pulmonary nodule ranges between 2.5 and 8.0, the lesion may be benign or malignant, and a comprehensive evaluation using combination methods with high-resolution computed tomography (HRCT) is recommended [27]. However, radiological signs associated with malignancy such as specular radiation, notching, and pleural indentation are also frequently manifested in tuberculoma on a CT scan as part of FDG PET/CT [28]. Sometimes, pulmonary lesions that cannot be diagnosed in terms of its malignancy on FDG PET scan could be successfully evaluated using other tracers, such as choline or somatostatin analog radiopharmaceuticals [29]. FDG PET/CT also shows low accuracy in the evaluation of lymph nodes' involvement in lung cancer patients with parenchymal sequelae from previous TB (Fig. 10.2) [30]. Tuberculosis is mostly responsible for false positive in lymph node staging of non-small-cell lung cancer (NSCLC) patients, and semiquantitative SUV method does not result in better diagnostic accuracy than visual analysis of PET images [31]. Dual-phase FDG PET imaging has been explored as a tool for the differentiation of inflammatory lesions from malignancy with some promising results. FDG uptake in inflammatory tissues reaches its peak in about 60 min after injection, but then it gradually decreases with time [32]. In tumors, an increased ratio of hexokinase/glucose-6-phosphatase may cause gradual accumulation of FDG and increase of SUV on delayed imaging. Conversely, high levels of glucose-6-phosphatase with rapid clearance of FDG and a low ratio of hexokinase to glucose-6-phosphatase are found in mononuclear cells, which represent the majority of cells in chronic inflammations [25]. Unfortunately, the studies which investigated this topic suggest that in patients presenting with solitary pulmonary nodule in area with high TB prevalence, dual-time FDG PET is unable to distinguish malignancy from TB, and further increase of FDG uptake with positive retention index is usually seen both in tuberculous and malignant lesions [25, 33]. Dual-time-point imaging with retention index also does not improve diagnostic accuracy of FDG PET/CT in lymph node staging of NSCLC patients, with TB as main cause of false-positive results [31]. These results also may indicate that other inflammatory cells or *Mycobacterium tuberculosis* itself could be the cause of high and increasing accumulation of FDG in tuberculomas over time, since it is shown that high levels of glucose are required for *M. tuberculosis* to construct their mycobacterial wall [25].

When comparing pulmonary tuberculous lesions with non-TB mycobacteriosis on FDG PET/CT, opposite results were reported regarding the degree of FDG uptake [34, 35], rendering thus this method ineffective in discriminating pulmonary infections caused by different mycobacterium species. No significant differences can be seen also with regard to CT features in patients with SPNs caused by *M. tuberculosis* or by mycobacterium avium complex (MAC) and their location or the presence of calcification, cavitation, central low attenuation, and satellite lesions [36]. On the other hand, nonspecific inflammatory nodules have significantly lower metabolism compared to tuberculous and malignant nodules [25, 26].

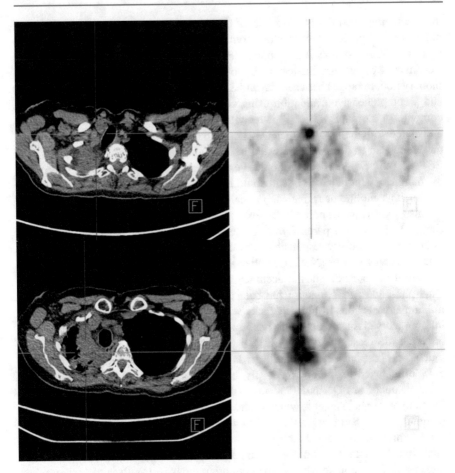

Fig. 10.2 Patient with right-upper lobectomy due to lung adenocarcinoma and atypical resection of superior segment of right-lower lobe due to TB, presenting with consolidation in apical parts of the remaining right lung with SUVmax 7.1 and high activity in right supraclavicular lymph node with SUVmax 9.2; FDG PET/CT is unable to differentiate between malignancy and active TB

It was already shown that FGD PET/CT has an important role in assessing activity of pulmonary and extrapulmonary TB lesions [37, 38]. However, there are still some difficulties in evaluation of disease activity and therapy response on FDG PET/CT. When FDG PET/CT was used in patients with no symptoms and symptomatic patients who had culturable TB, SUVmax was in the same range [39]. Increased FDG uptake on PET/CT has been reported in old TB lesions and in patients following treatment after a clinical cure without developing disease during follow-up [37, 40, 41]. This does not necessarily suggest active disease and may be the effect of an equilibrium state between the host immune system and replicating bacilli. During treatment monitoring, some lesions can be more active on follow-up than on the initial scan or new lesions could appear in patients who achieved and sustained a clinical cure. These new TB lesions could be explained by different responses of various TB lesions and microevolution in subpopulations of *M. tuberculosis*. However, there are still no clear guidelines on interpretation of mixed response [42]. Therefore, FDG PET/CT scan must be interpreted not solely based on metabolic activity of the lesion, but by taking the patient's clinical presentation into account and also correlating metabolic uptake with CT findings.

In patients with human immunodeficiency virus (HIV) and TB coinfection, lesions may appear to be in progression following initiation of antiretroviral therapy while on tuberculostatics, which may be explained as inflammation caused by immune reconstitution with increased FDG uptake, and that should not be misinterpreted as poor response to therapy on FDG PET/CT study [43]. Another cause of pitfalls on FDG PET/CT imaging is that radiographic appearance of TB can be confused with co-pathologies of the lung frequently seen in HIV-infected individuals, such as *Pneumocystis jirovecii* pneumonia or nontuberculous mycobacterium infections; bacterial, fungal, or viral pneumonia; Kaposi sarcoma or non-Hodgkin lymphoma [44], etc. There is also a question regarding the specificity of FDG in HIV-positive patients with TB and lymphoma, and although the mean splenic metabolic uptake is increased in HIV patients with lymphoma compared to those with reactive adenopathy, this finding would most likely overlap between TB and lymphoma [44, 45].

On FDG PET/CT, the increased uptake in lymph nodes associated with active TB can be indistinguishable from other causes of FDG-avid lymphadenopathies, such as lymphoma (Fig. 10.3) [18, 19, 46] or sarcoidosis [47]. Lymphadenopathy, fever, weakness, night sweats, and weight loss are all common clinical presentations of lymph node tuberculosis (LNTB), causing a notable risk of confusing LNTB with lymphomas [48]. FDG PET is not able differentiate malignant lymph node involvement from LNTB, with no significant difference between the median SUVmean values of involved lymph node basins [49]. On the other hand, sarcoidosis and TB, the two most common benign causes of mediastinal lymphadenopathy, also share

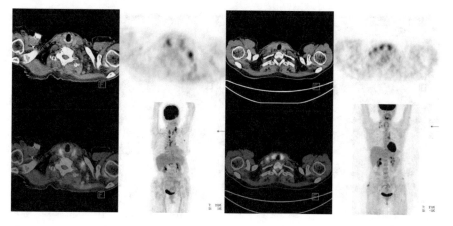

Fig. 10.3 On the left, patient with lymph node tuberculosis, on the right Hodgkin lymphoma patient

remarkable clinical, radiologic, and histologic similarities, with also a myriad of nonspecific manifestation of sarcoidosis seen on FDG PET/CT not different from TB itself [50, 51]. The pattern of FDG uptake in various lymph node groups of the body, percentage of patients with pulmonary parenchymal FDG positivity and patterns of FDG uptake in the lung parenchyma, and in affected extrapulmonary organs show similarities in patients with TB and sarcoidosis (Fig. 10.4). There is also no difference in both early and delayed SUVmax between TB and sarcoidosis, with most of the patients showing positive retention index, which all indicates futility of this imaging modality in differentiation of these two entities [47].

When evaluating pleural effusion, metabolic activity alone is not enough to distinguish TB from malignant causes [52, 53]. Although sometimes the addition of morphological CT findings to PET uptake pattern can improve specificity, there are some patterns on FDG PET/CT typical for malignancies that can be also seen in TB, which could lead to falsely characterizing the effusion as malignant, such as no pleural thickening with multiple nodular FDG uptake, nodular pleural thickening with nodular FDG uptake, and irregular pleural thickening with diffuse FDG uptake (Fig. 10.5) [54].

Myocardial TB involvement may be difficult to discern due to physiological FDG uptake, and dietary preparations in order to reduce physiological myocardial FDG uptake are recommended [55].

High physiologic uptake of FDG in the brain may decrease the sensitivity of the detection of central nervous system TB lesions. There is also a problem of prednisolone use before the PET scan, as corticosteroid administration may result in membrane stabilization, reduced inflammation, and increased blood sugar level, which may attenuate FDG uptake leading to false-negative result, and thus reduce sensitivity of FDG PET/CT in revealing cranial lesions by up to 30% when compared to MRI [56].

Clinical presentation of abdominal TB is usually nonspecific and related to the affected area, so it may be difficult to diagnose. Peritoneal tuberculosis can mimic

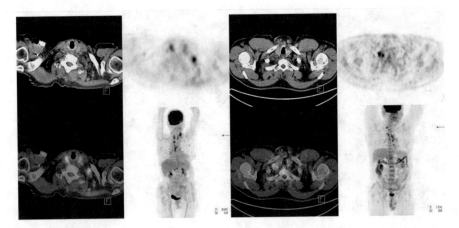

Fig. 10.4 Left image—patient with TB lymphadenitis, right image—patient with sarcoidosis

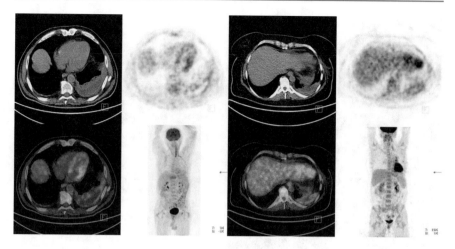

Fig. 10.5 Image on the left showing patient with tuberculous pleuritis; image on the right displaying pleural involvement in patient with lung cancer

peritoneal carcinomatosis (PC), sometimes with elevated serum CA125 levels, and showing even increase in FDG uptake on delayed images [21, 57–59]. In both peritoneal thickening and ascites, discrimination between TB and malignant peritoneal involvement on FDG PET/CT is more challenging compared with other benign causes of peritoneal disease [60, 61]. There is no difference in metabolic activity between tuberculous peritonitis (TBP) and PC, and although extensive involvement, uniform distribution, string-of-beads sign, and smooth uniform thickening might be significant differential features of TBP [62], pathological proof is often required. Nonspecific intestinal FDG uptake can cause a practical problem in PET images interpretation when digestive system TB is suspected. Although uptake pattern in the intestine can be focal even in cases of intraluminal secretion, it may change with time, and a delayed image may be useful to distinguish the physiologic intestinal uptake from pathologic one. There are some reports of high metabolic activity seen on FDG PET/CT in stomach, duodenum, jejunum, and colon initially suspected to be malignant, some of which even showed further increase of uptake on delayed images, but finally tuberculous etiology was proved [15, 63–65]. Hepatic TB has been shown to may mimic intrahepatic cholangiocarcinoma on FDG PET/CT [66] or metastatic disease (Fig. 10.6). Solitary spleen TB has been described on FDG PET/CT mimicking melanoma deposit [9]. On the other hand, micronodular hepatosplenic involvement, characterized by innumerable small nodules with irregular ill-defined margins, could be missed on FDG PET/CT [67].

In disease that affects the organs involved in excretion of FDG, such as the kidney, bladder, or urinary tract, FDG PET/CT demonstrates poor sensitivity and should be complemented with other imaging modalities such as contrast enhanced CT/CT urography to confirm results and minimize false-negative findings [67]. Sometimes focal increased uptake corresponding to a renal nodule can be identified on FDG-PET/CT in cases of renal TB, but this finding is nonspecific and may mimic

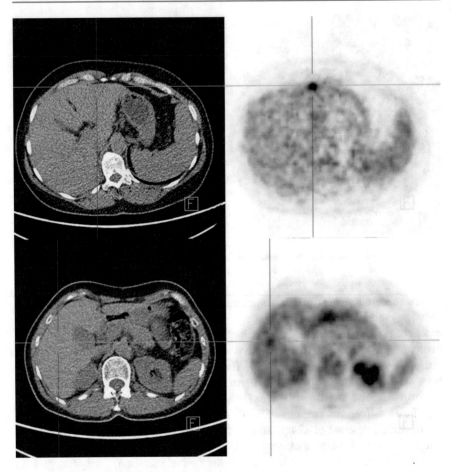

Fig. 10.6 Focal lesion in the liver—top row patient with tuberculous liver involvement; bottom row liver metastasis in patient with colorectal carcinoma

renal cell carcinoma, although dual-time-point imaging may be useful for defining the TB lesions [16, 22].

Physiological uterine and ovarian uptake in women must be taken into account during evaluation of disease status, and unilateral increased ovarian FDG uptake can be functional in non-menopausal patients. To confirm the ovarian localization of the disease, patients should undergo additional evaluation, such as magnetic resonance imaging or laparoscopy [68]. With regard to musculoskeletal tuberculosis, there are cases in literature where skeletal TB was initially mistaken for disseminated metastatic disease on FDG PET/CT, particularly when presented with atypical features [69–71].

Less common sites of TB detected on FDG PET/CT described in literature, which could be perplexing to interpret and often mimic other inflammatory and particularly malignant diseases, include pharyngeal and laryngeal TB, tuberculosis of esophagus, tuberculous myocarditis, TB of the breast, adrenal TB, tuberculosis of common bile duct, prostate and epididymis TB, skin erythema nodosum due to TB, and anal fistula caused by TB [17, 72–81].

References

1. Ramos JP, Batista MV, Costa SF. Tuberculosis in hematopoietic stem cell transplant recipients. Mediterr J Hematol Infect Dis. 2013;5:e201306. https://doi.org/10.4084/MJHID.2013.061.
2. Simonsen DF, Farkas DK, Horsburgh CR, Thomsen RW, Sørensen HT. Increased risk of active tuberculosis after cancer diagnosis. J Infect. 2017;74:590–8. https://doi.org/10.1016/j.jinf.2017.03.012.
3. Huebner RE, Schein MF, Bass JB Jr. The tuberculin skin test. Clin Infect Dis. 1993;17:968–75.
4. Shiels MS, Albanes D, Virtamo J, Engels EA. Increased risk of lung cancer in men with tuberculosis in the alpha-tocopherol, beta-carotene cancer prevention study. Cancer Epidemiol Biomark Prev. 2011;20:672–8. https://doi.org/10.1158/1055-9965.EPI-10-1166.
5. Huber H, Hodolic M, Stelzmüller I, Wunn R, Hatzl M, Fellner F, et al. Malignant disease as an incidental finding at ^{18}F-FDG-PET/CT scanning in patients with granulomatous lung disease. Nucl Med Commun. 2015;36:430–7. https://doi.org/10.1097/MNM.0000000000000274.
6. Sobic-Saranovic D, Petrusic I, Artiko V, Pavlovic S, Subotic D, Saranovic D, Nagorni-Obradovic L, Petrovic N, Todorovic-Tirnanic M, Odalovic S, Grozdic-Milojevic I, Stoiljkovic M, Obradovic V. Comparison of 18F-FDG PET/CT and MDCT for staging/restaging of non-small cell lung cancer. Neoplasma. 2015;62:295–301. https://doi.org/10.4149/neo_2015_035.
7. Ando M, Mukai Y, Ushijima RI, Shioyama Y, Umeki K, Okada F, et al. Disseminated Mycobacterium tuberculosis infection masquerading as metastasis after heavy ion radiotherapy for prostate cancer. Intern Med. 2016;55:3387–92. https://doi.org/10.2169/internalmedicine.55.7039.
8. Bhattacharya A, Agrawal KL, Kashyap R, Manohar K, Mittal BR, Varma SC, et al. Coexisting tuberculosis and non-Hodgkin's lymphoma on 18F-Fluorodeoxyglucose PET-CT. J Postgrad Med Educ Res. 2012;46:49–50. https://doi.org/10.5005/jp-journals-10028-1012.
9. Cegla P, Spychala A, Marszalek A, Wierzchoslawska E, Cholewinski W. Atypical spleen tuberculosis in a melanoma patient accidentally detected during a (18)F-FDG PET/CT study: case report. Mol Clin Oncol. 2018;8:89–92. https://doi.org/10.3892/mco.2017.1498.
10. Chaudhary P, Gupta S, Leekha N, Rajendra RS, Mishra SS, Arora V, et al. Ambiguity of whole body PET CT scans in diagnosis of co-existing tuberculosis and malignancy: is histopathological confirmation mandatory? Gulf J Oncolog. 2017;1:15–9.
11. Chen C, Zhu YH, Qian HY, Huang JA. Pulmonary tuberculosis with false-positive (18) F-fluorodeoxyglucose positron emission tomography mimicking recurrent lung cancer: a case report. Exp Ther Med. 2015;9:159–61. https://doi.org/10.3892/etm.2014.2054.
12. D'souza MM, Mondal A, Sharma R, Jaimini A, Khanna U. Tuberculosis the great mimicker: 18F-fludeoxyglucose positron emission tomography/computed tomography in a case of atypical spinal tuberculosis. Indian J Nucl Med. 2014;29:99–101. https://doi.org/10.4103/0972-3919.130294.
13. Harkirat S, Anana SS, Indrajit LK, Dash AK. Pictorial essay: PET/CT in tuberculosis. Indian J Radiol Imaging. 2008;18:141–7. https://doi.org/10.4103/0971-3026.40299.
14. Hofmeyr A, Lau WF, Slavin MA. Mycobacterium tuberculosis infection in patients with cancer, the role of 18-fluorodeoxyglucose positron emission tomography for diagnosis and monitoring treatment response. Tuberculosis (Edinb). 2007;87:459–63. https://doi.org/10.1016/j.tube.2007.05.013.
15. Jehanno N, Cassou-Mounat T, Vincent-Salomon A, Luporsi M, Bedoui M, Kuhnowski F. PET/CT imaging in management of concomitant Hodgkin lymphoma and tuberculosis—a problem solver tool. Clin Case Rep. 2017;6:232–4. https://doi.org/10.1002/ccr3.1248.

16. Kamaleshwaran K, Shinto A, Natarajan S, Mohanan V. F-18 FDG PET/CT in tuberculosis: non-invasive marker of therapeutic response to Antitubercular therapy. Int J Nucl. 2015;2:22–4. https://doi.org/10.15379/2408-9788.2015.02.01.5.
17. Lee G, Lee JH, Park SG. F-18 FDG PET/CT imaging of solitary genital tuberculosis mimicking recurrent lymphoma. Clin Nucl Med. 2011;36:315–6. https://doi.org/10.1097/RLU.0b013e31820aa033.
18. Mukherjee A, Sharma P, Karunanithi S, Dhull VS, Kumar R. Lymphoma and tuberculosis: temporal evolution of dual pathology on sequential 18F-FDG PET/CT. Clin Nucl Med. 2014;39:736–7. https://doi.org/10.1097/RLU.0000000000000368.
19. Omri HE, Hascsi Z, Taha R, Szabados L, Sabah HE, Gamiel A, et al. Tubercular meningitis and lymphadenitis mimicking a relapse of Burkitt's lymphoma on (18)F-FDG-PET/CT: a case report. Case Rep Oncol. 2015;8:226–32. https://doi.org/10.1159/000430768.
20. Sengul A, Arslan S, Tasolar F, Kapicibasi O. Coexistence of lung cancer and primary lymph nodes tuberculosis diagnosed by cancer staging: a report of a rare case. Ann Clin Case Rep. 2016;1:1136.
21. Shimamoto H, Hamada K, Higuchi I, Tsujihata M, Nonomura N, Tomita Y, et al. Abdominal tuberculosis: peritoneal involvement shown by F-18 FDG PET. Clin Nucl Med. 2007;32:716–8. https://doi.org/10.1097/RLU.0b013e318123f813.
22. Subramanyam P, Palaniswamy SS. Dual time point (18)F-FDG PET/CT imaging identifies bilateral renal tuberculosis in an immunocompromised patient with an unknown primary malignancy. Infect Chemother. 2015;47:117–9. https://doi.org/10.3947/ic.2015.47.2.117.
23. Wakasugi M, Tanemura M, Mikami T, Furukawa K, Tsujimoto M, Akamatsu H. Liver hilar tuberculous lymphadenitis successfully diagnosed by laparoscopic lymph node biopsy. Int J Surg Case Rep. 2015;10:191–4. https://doi.org/10.1016/j.ijscr.2015.03.002.
24. Li Y, Su M, Li F, Kuang A, Tian R. The value of 18F FDG-PET/CT in the differential diagnosis of solitary pulmonary nodules in areas with high incidence of tuberculosis. Ann Nucl Med. 2011;25:804–11. https://doi.org/10.1007/s12149-011-0530-y.
25. Sathekge MM, Maes A, Pottel H, Stoltz A, van de Wiele C. Dual time-point FDG PET-CT for differentiating benign from malignant solitary pulmonary nodules in a TB endemic area. S Afr Med J. 2010;100:598–601. https://doi.org/10.7196/SAMJ.4082.
26. Purandare NC, Pramesh CS, Agarwal JP, Agrawal A, Shah S, Prabhash K, et al. Solitary pulmonary nodule evaluation in regions endemic for infectious diseases: do regional variations impact the effectiveness of fluorodeoxyglucose positron emission tomography/computed tomography. Indian J Cancer. 2017;54:271–5. https://doi.org/10.4103/0019-509X.219563.
27. Hou S, Lin X, Wang S, Shen Y, Meng Z, Jia Q, et al. Combination of positron emission tomography/computed tomography and chest thin-layer high-resolution computed tomography for evaluation of pulmonary nodules: correlation with imaging features, maximum standardized uptake value, and pathology. Medicine (Baltimore). 2018;97:e11640. https://doi.org/10.1097/MD.0000000000011640.
28. Zheng Z, Pan Y, Guo F, Wei H, Wu S, Pan T, et al. Multimodality FDG PET/CT appearance of pulmonary tuberculoma mimicking lung cancer and pathologic correlation in a tuberculosis-endemic country. South Med J. 2011;104:440–5. https://doi.org/10.1097/SMJ.0b013e318218700a.
29. Sobic-Saranovic DP, Pavlovic SV, Artiko VM, Saranovic DZ, Jaksic ED, Subotic D, Nagorni-Obradovic L, Kozarevic N, Petrovic N, Grozdic IT, Obradovic VB. The utility of two somatostatin analog radiopharmaceuticals in assessment of radiologically indeterminate pulmonary lesions. Clin Nucl Med. 2012;37:14–20. https://doi.org/10.1097/RLU.0b013e3182335edb.
30. Lee SH, Min JW, Lee CH, Park CM, Goo JM, Chung DH, et al. Impact of parenchymal tuberculosis sequelae on mediastinal lymph node staging in patients with lung cancer. J Korean Med Sci. 2011;26:67–70. https://doi.org/10.3346/jkms.2011.26.1.67.
31. Yen RF, Chen KC, Lee JM, Chang YC, Wang J, Cheng MF, et al. 18F-FDG PET for the lymph node staging of non-small cell lung cancer in a tuberculosis-endemic country: is dual time point imaging worth the effort? Eur J Nucl Med Mol Imaging. 2008;35:1305–15. https://doi.org/10.1007/s00259-008-0733-1.

32. Yamada S, Kubota K, Kubota R, Ido T, Tamahashi N. High accumulation of Fluorine-18-Fluorodeoxyglucose in turpentine-induced inflammatory tissue. J Nucl Med. 1995;36:1301–6.

33. Chen CJ, Lee BF, Yao WJ, Cheng L, Wu PS, Chu CL, et al. Dual-phase 18F-FDG PET in the diagnosis of pulmonary nodules with an initial standard uptake value less than 2.5. AJR Am J Roentgenol. 2008;191:475–9. https://doi.org/10.2214/AJR.07.3457.

34. Del Giudice G, Bianco A, Cennamo A, Santoro G, Bifulco M, Marzo C, et al. Lung and nodal involvement in Nontuberculous mycobacterial disease: PET/CT role. Biomed Res Int. 2015;2015:353202. https://doi.org/10.1155/2015/353202.

35. Demura Y, Tsuchida T, Uesaka D, Umeda Y, Morikawa M, Ameshima S, et al. Usefulness of 18F-fluorodeoxyglucose positron emission tomography for diagnosing disease activity and monitoring therapeutic response in patients with pulmonary mycobacteriosis. Eur J Nucl Med Mol Imaging. 2009;36:632–9. https://doi.org/10.1007/s00259-008-1009-5.

36. Hahm CR, Park HY, Jeon K, Um SW, Suh GY, Chung MP, et al. Solitary pulmonary nodules caused by mycobacterium tuberculosis and Mycobacterium avium complex. Lung. 2010;188:25–31. https://doi.org/10.1007/s00408-009-9203-1.

37. Heysell SK, Thomas TA, Sifri CD, Rehm PK, Houpt ER. 18-Fluorodeoxyglucose positron emission tomography for tuberculosis diagnosis and management: a case series. BMC Pulm Med. 2013;13:14. https://doi.org/10.1186/1471-2466-13-14.

38. Kim IJ, Lee JS, Kim SJ, Kim YK, Jeong YJ, Jun S, et al. Double-phase 18F-FDG PET-CT for determination of pulmonary tuberculoma activity. Eur J Nucl Med Mol Imaging. 2008;35:808–14. https://doi.org/10.1007/s00259-007-0585-0.

39. Geadas C, Acuna-Villaorduna C, Mercier G, Kleinman MB, Horsburgh CR Jr, Ellner JJ, et al. FDG-PET/CT activity leads to the diagnosis of unsuspected TB: a retrospective study. BMC Res Notes. 2018;11:464. https://doi.org/10.1186/s13104-018-3564-6.

40. Jeong YJ, Paeng JC, Nam HY, Lee JS, Lee SM, Yoo CG, et al. (18)F-FDG positron-emission tomography/computed tomography findings of radiographic lesions suggesting old healed tuberculosis. J Korean Med Sci. 2014;29:386–91. https://doi.org/10.3346/jkms.2014.29.3.386.

41. Malherbe ST, Shenai S, Ronacher K, Loxton AG, Dolganov G, Kriel M, et al. Persisting positron emission tomography lesion activity and Mycobacterium tuberculosis mRNA after tuberculosis cure. Nat Med. 2016;22:1094–100. https://doi.org/10.1038/nm.4177.

42. Sathekge MM, Ankrah AO, Lawal I, Vorster M. Monitoring response to therapy. Semin Nucl Med. 2018;48:166–81. https://doi.org/10.1053/j.semnuclmed.2017.10.004.

43. Ankrah AO, Glaudemans AWJM, Maes A, Van de Wiele C, Dierckx RAJO, Vorster M, et al. Tuberculosis. Semin Nucl Med. 2018;48:108–30. https://doi.org/10.1053/j.semnuclmed.2017.10.005.

44. Sathekge M, Maes A, Van de Wiele C. FDG-PET imaging in HIV infection and tuberculosis. Semin Nucl Med. 2013;43:349–66. https://doi.org/10.1053/j.semnuclmed.2013.04.008.

45. Sathekge M. Differentiation of HIV-associated lymphoma from HIV-reactive adenopathy using quantitative FDG-PET and symmetry. Eur J Nucl Med Mol Imaging. 2014;41:593–5. https://doi.org/10.1007/s00259-014-2701-2.

46. Ouedraogo M, Ouedraogo SM, Cisse R, Lougue C, Badoum G, Sigani A, et al. Active tuberculosis in a patient with Hodgkin's disease. A case report. Rev Pneumol Clin. 2000;56:33–5.

47. Maturu VN, Agarwal R, Aggarwal AN, Mittal BR, Bal A, Gupta N, et al. Dual-time point whole-body 18F-fluorodeoxyglucose PET/CT imaging in undiagnosed mediastinal lymphadenopathy: a prospective study of 117 patients with sarcoidosis and TB. Chest. 2014;146:e216–20. https://doi.org/10.1378/chest.14-1827.

48. Ding RL, Cao HY, Hu Y, Shang CL, Xie F, Zhang ZH, et al. Lymph node tuberculosis mimicking malignancy on (18)F-FDG PET/CT in two patients: a case report. Exp Ther Med. 2017;13:3369–73. https://doi.org/10.3892/etm.2017.4421.

49. Sathekge M, Maes A, Kgomo M, Pottel H, Stolz A, Van De Wiele C. FDG uptake in lymph-nodes of HIV+ and tuberculosis patients: implications for cancer staging. Q J Nucl Med Mol Imaging. 2010;54:698–703.

50. Gupta D, Agarwal R, Aggarwal AN, Jindal SK. Sarcoidosis and tuberculosis: the same disease with different manifestations or similar manifestations of different disorders. Curr Opin Pulm Med. 2012;18:506–16. https://doi.org/10.1097/MCP.0b013e3283560809.

51. Sobic-Saranovic D, Artiko V, Obradovic V. FDG PET imaging in sarcoidosis. Semin Nucl Med. 2013;43:404–11. https://doi.org/10.1053/j.semnuclmed.2013.06.007.

52. Orki A, Akin O, Tasci AE, Ciftci H, Urek S, Falay O, et al. The role of positron emission tomography/computed tomography in the diagnosis of pleural diseases. Thorac Cardiovasc Surg. 2009;57:217–21. https://doi.org/10.1055/s-2008-1039314.

53. Shinohara T, Shiota N, Kume M, Hamada N, Naruse K, Ogushi F. Asymptomatic primary tuberculous pleurisy with intense 18-fluorodeoxyglucose uptake mimicking malignant mesothelioma. BMC Infect Dis. 2013;13:12. https://doi.org/10.1186/1471-2334-13-12.

54. Sun Y, Yu H, Ma J, Lu P. The role of 18F-FDG PET/CT integrated imaging in distinguishing malignant from benign pleural effusion. PLoS One. 2016;11:e0161764. https://doi.org/10.1371/journal.pone.0161764.

55. Osborne MT, Hulten EA, Murthy VL, Skali H, Taqueti VR, Dorbala S, et al. Patient preparation for cardiac fluorine-18 fluorodeoxyglucose positron emission tomography imaging of inflammation. J Nucl Cardiol. 2017;24:86–99. https://doi.org/10.1007/s12350-016-0502-7.

56. Gambhir S, Kumar M, Ravina M, Bhoi SK, Kalita J, Misra UK. Role of (18)F-FDG PET in demonstrating disease burden in patients with tuberculous meningitis. J Neurol Sci. 2016;370:196–200. https://doi.org/10.1016/j.jns.2016.09.051.

57. Chen CJ, Yao WJ, Chou CY, Chiu NT, Lee BF, Wu PS. Peritoneal tuberculosis with elevated serum CA125 mimicking peritoneal carcinomatosis on F-18 FDG-PET/CT. Ann Nucl Med. 2008;22:525–7. https://doi.org/10.1007/s12149-008-0139-y.

58. Koc S, Beydilli G, Tulunay G, Ocalan R, Boran N, Ozgul N, et al. Peritoneal tuberculosis mimicking advanced ovarian cancer: a retrospective review of 22 cases. Gynecol Oncol. 2006;103:565–9. https://doi.org/10.1016/j.ygyno.2006.04.010.

59. Takalkar AM, Bruno GL, Reddy M, Lilien DL. Intense FDG activity in peritoneal tuberculosis mimics peritoneal carcinomatosis. Clin Nucl Med. 2007;32:244–6. https://doi.org/10.1097/01.rlu.0000255239.04475.c2.

60. Chen R, Chen Y, Liu L, Zhou X, Liu J, Huang G. The role of ^{18}F-FDG PET/CT in the evaluation of peritoneal thickening of undetermined origin. Medicine (Baltimore). 2016;95:e3023. https://doi.org/10.1097/MD.0000000000003023.

61. Zhang M, Jiang X, Zhang M, Xu H, Zhai G, Li B. The role of 18F-FDG PET/CT in the evaluation of ascites of undetermined origin. J Nucl Med. 2009;50:506–12. https://doi.org/10.2967/jnumed.108.056382.

62. Wang SB, Ji YH, Wu HB, Wang QS, Zhou WL, Lv L, et al. PET/CT for differentiating between tuberculous peritonitis and peritoneal carcinomatosis: the parietal peritoneum. Medicine (Baltimore). 2017;96:e5867. https://doi.org/10.1097/MD.0000000000005867.

63. Akdogan RA, Halil Rakici AA, Güngör S, Bedir R, Akdogan E. F-18 Fluorodeoxyglucose positron emission tomography/computed tomography findings of isolated gastric tuberculosis mimicking gastric cancer and lymphoma. Euroasian J Hepatogastroenterol. 2018;8:93–6. https://doi.org/10.5005/jp-journals-10018-1270.

64. Jung JH, Kim SH, Kim MJ, Cho YK, Ahn SB, Son BK, et al. A case report of primary duodenal tuberculosis mimicking a malignant tumor. Clin Endosc. 2014;47:346–9. https://doi.org/10.5946/ce.2014.47.4.346.

65. Wang HY, Lin WY. Jejunal tuberculosis: incidental finding on an FDG-PET scan. Kaohsiung J Med Sci. 2006;22:34–8. https://doi.org/10.1016/S1607-551X(09)70218-9.

66. Park JI. Primary hepatic tuberculosis mimicking intrahepatic cholangiocarcinoma: report of two cases. Ann Surg Treat Res. 2015;89:98–101. https://doi.org/10.4174/astr.2015.89.2.98.

67. Ito K, Morooka M, Minamimoto R, Miyata Y, Okasaki M, Kubota K. Imaging spectrum and pitfalls of ^{18}F-fluorodeoxyglucose positron emission tomography/computed tomography in patients with tuberculosis. Jpn J Radiol. 2013;31:511–20. https://doi.org/10.1007/s11604-013-0218-4.

68. Martinez V, Castilla-Lievre MA, Guillet-Caruba C, Grenier G, Fior R, Desarnaud S, et al. (18) F-FDG PET/CT in tuberculosis: an early non-invasive marker of therapeutic response. Int J Tuberc Lung Dis. 2012;16:1180–5. https://doi.org/10.5588/ijtld.12.0010.
69. Cho YS, Chung DR, Lee EJ, Kim BT, Lee KH. 18F-FDG PET/CT in a case of multifocal skeletal tuberculosis without pulmonary disease and potential role for monitoring treatment response. Clin Nucl Med. 2014;39:980–3. https://doi.org/10.1097/RLU.0000000000000363.
70. Go SW, Lee HY, Lim CH, Jee WH, Wang YP, Yoo IR, et al. Atypical disseminated skeletal tuberculosis mimicking metastasis on PET-CT and MRI. Intern Med. 2012;51:2961–5. https://doi.org/10.2169/internalmedicine.51.8347.
71. Liu B, Dong L, Wang X, Han T, Lin Q, Liu M. Tuberculosis mimicking metastases by malignancy in FDG PET/CT. QJM. 2017;110:173–4. https://doi.org/10.1093/qjmed/hcw214.
72. Bakheet SM, Powe J, Kandil A, Ezzat A, Rostom A, Amartey J. F-18 FDG uptake in breast infection and inflammation. Clin Nucl Med. 2000;25:100–3. https://doi.org/10.1097/00003072-200002000-00003.
73. Cengiz A, Göksel S, Başal Y, Taş Gülen Ş, Döğer F, Yürekli Y. Laryngeal tuberculosis mimicking laryngeal carcinoma on (18)F-FDG PET/CT imaging. Mol Imaging Radionucl Ther. 2018;27:81–3. https://doi.org/10.1097/RLU.0000000000000656.
74. Chen X, Lu H, Gao Y. FDG PET/CT showing erythema nodosum associated with tuberculous lymphadenitis. Clin Nucl Med. 2013;38:992–3. https://doi.org/10.1097/RLU.0000000000000233.
75. Das CJ, Kumar R, Balakrishnan VB, Chawla M, Malhotra A. Disseminated tuberculosis masquerading as metastatic breast carcinoma on PET-CT. Clin Nucl Med. 2008;33:359–61. https://doi.org/10.1097/RLU.0b013e31816a858e.
76. Dong A, Wang Y, Gong J, Zuo C. FDG PET/CT findings of common bile duct tuberculosis. Clin Nucl Med. 2013;39:67–70. https://doi.org/10.1097/RLU.0b013e318279c170.
77. Garg G, Tripathi M, D'Souza M, Jaimini A, Jain N, Khurana A, et al. Demonstration of a tubercular fistula-in-ano on F-18 FDG PET/CT. Clin Nucl Med. 2010;35:300–2. https://doi.org/10.1097/RLU.0b013e3181d18ccb.
78. Ito K, Morooka M, Kubota K. 18F-FDG PET/CT findings of pharyngeal tuberculosis. Ann Nucl Med. 2010;24:493–6. https://doi.org/10.1007/s12149-010-0368-8.
79. Kadihasanoglu M, Yildiz T, Atahan S, Ausmus A, Atahan O. 18F-flouro-2-deoxyglucose positron emission tomography/computed tomography imaging of solitary prostatic and pulmonary tuberculosis mimicking metastatic prostate cancer. J Cancer Res Ther. 2015;11:663. https://doi.org/10.4103/0973-1482.143354.
80. Roudaut N, Malecot JM, Dupont E, Boussion N, Visvikis D, Doucet L, et al. Adrenal tuberculosis revealed by FDG PET. Clin Nucl Med. 2008;33:821–3. https://doi.org/10.1097/RLU.0b013e318187ee60.
81. Sperry BW, Oldan JD, Hsich EM, Reynolds JP, Tamarappoo BK. Infectious myocarditis on FDG-PET imaging mimicking Sarcoidosis. J Nucl Cardiol. 2015;22:840–4. https://doi.org/10.1007/s12350-015-0160-1.

FDG-PET in Treatment Response Assessment of Tuberculosis

11

I. O. Lawal and Mike Sathekge

Contents

11.1 Introduction

Treatment of tuberculosis (TB) involves the use of multiple drugs for an extended period of time. In the treatment of drug-sensitive pulmonary TB (PTB), therapy is administered for 6 months, whereas extrapulmonary TB (EPTB) is usually treated for longer. In multidrug resistance TB (MDR-TB), treatment is continued for 18–24 months after sputum conversion. This long duration of TB treatment with multiple drugs exposes patients to potential side effects, increases the chances of drug–drug interactions, treatment nonadherence, and the development of drug resistance [1–3]. On an economic scale, TB treatment places a high burden on the public health system [4, 5]. Several efforts are being made to address some of these challenges associated with TB care, such as shortening the duration of treatment [6]. In patients with drug-sensitive TB (DR-TB) treated with a standard regimen of first-line therapy, less than 5% will experience relapse [7]. On the contrary, about 20% of

I. O. Lawal (✉) · M. Sathekge
Department of Nuclear Medicine, University of Pretoria & Steve Biko Academic Hospital, Pretoria, South Africa
e-mail: mike.sathekge@up.ac.za

© Springer Nature Switzerland AG 2020
D. Sobic Saranovic et al. (eds.), *PET/CT in Tuberculosis*, Clinicians' Guides to Radionuclide Hybrid Imaging, https://doi.org/10.1007/978-3-030-47009-8_11

patients treated with short-course regimen lasting 4 months experience relapse [8]. This, therefore, suggests that some patients may experience sterilizing cure with a regimen shorter than the standard 6 months. Treatment response assessment to identify early responders is crucial to determine patients who may benefit from shorter treatment duration and to assess the adequacy of treatment.

Response to TB treatment is traditionally assessed using sputum smear and culture at 2 and 6 months after initiation of therapy. Both of these techniques have several limitations in their abilities to predict durable cure. Sputum smear, though cheap and widely available, is poorly sensitive particularly when the bacillary load is reduced by treatment, is operator-dependent, cannot differentiate live from dead bacteria, cannot reliably differentiate *Mycobacterium tuberculosis* from nontuberculous mycobacteria and is a poor predictor of treatment outcome [9–11]. Mycobacterial culture is time-consuming, prone to contamination, is expensive, and not readily available in TB-endemic communities [12, 13]. Blood-borne inflammatory markers such as erythrocyte sedimentation rate and C-reactive protein are nonspecific for TB [14]. Several novel biomarkers have been tested for their ability to assess response to anti-TB treatment (ATT) [15]. CD4 + T-cells play a crucial role in fighting TB infection. CD4 + cells secrete gamma interferon (IFN-γ). T-cell-based IFN-γ released assays (IGRAs) provide an objective measure to assess the function of T-cells. Most patients with TB are IGRA-positive, about 10–20% of patients, however, have a negative or indeterminate IFN-γ response to TB antigen stimulation [16]. Similarly, depletion of CD4+ T-cells in individuals with human immunodeficiency virus (HIV) infection also makes this test less reliable in them. Xpert MTB/RIF assay is the World Health Organization (WHO)–approved sputum-based real-time polymerase chain reaction (PCR) method for rapid diagnosis of TB and for assessing sensitivity to Rifampicin. It also suffers from poor specificity as dead mycobacterial can cause false-positive assay [17].

Imaging is a useful modality for response assessment [18]. Chest X-ray (CXR), the most commonly used imaging modality for response assessment, has lower sensitivity and specificity compared with computed tomography (CT). Generally, morphologic imaging with either CT or MRI can be unreliable for response assessment due to the difficulty encountered sometimes in differentiating active from a healed inactive lesion at the completion of treatment. While TB lesions may resolve completely following therapy in some patients, residual lesions are often seen in others after successful treatment [19, 20]. In some cases, TB granulomas may increase in size despite sterilizing cure [18]. Residual lesions characterized as old, healed lesions on TB can sometimes contain slowly replicating or nonreplicating tubercle bacilli, the cause of relapse after treatment [20]. Also in EPTB, resolution of morphologic changes due to TB may lag sterilizing cure [21].

11.2 FDG-PET for Response Assessment

Hybrid imaging with F-18-labeled fluorodeoxyglucose (FDG) positron emission tomography/computed tomography (PET/CT), initially used in oncologic imaging, has gained popular application for imaging of inflammation and infection [22, 23].

The TB granuloma is abundant in macrophages [24]. Activated macrophages have enhanced glucose utilization to meet the energy requirement of the metabolically demanding protective immune function. FDG is an analog of glucose that is trapped similarly as glucose but does undergo further embolism in the glycolytic pathway after the initial phosphorylation. It is therefore metabolically trapped for PET imaging, with resultant intense FDG uptake in active TB lesions [18, 25, 26]. After a successful anti-TB treatment, sterilization of the granuloma leads to a cessation of the inflammatory response. Consequently, FDG uptake in sterilized granuloma returns to background level [27, 28]. FDG-PET/CT imaging offers a whole-body hybrid morphologic and metabolic assessment of PTB and EPTB response to treatment in one imaging session.

FDG-PET/CT imaging for response assessment has been done at different time points during ATT and at the completion of treatment. FDG-PET/CT imaging done during treatment may be useful to identify early response or lack of it (Fig. 11.1). Incorporating FDG-PET/CT imaging into TB treatment may prove helpful to determine the length of treatment and for individualization of therapy. Treatment duration, based on current recommendations, are largely empirical especially as it applies to the treatment of MDR-TB. Martinez et al. performed FDG-PET/CT for response assessment after 1 month of anti-TB therapy in a group of prospectively recruited patients with PTB and EPTB [29]. All but two patients in the study had a significant drop in the FDG uptake in TB lesions with a median decrease in maximum standardized uptake value (SUVmax) of 31% compared with a baseline FDG-PET/CT. One of the two patients with no demonstrable response on FDG-PET/CT was a case of non-Hodgkin lymphoma misdiagnosed as tuberculous lymphadenitis. This study shows the ability of FDG-PET/CT to determine response to treatment as early as after 1 month of treatment. Patients without demonstrable response based on FDG-PET findings may already be reviewed for adherence. As demonstrated in the patient misdiagnosed and treated for TB, alternative diagnosis may be considered when no response to a trial of ATT is seen especially when the initial diagnosis is probably [29].

FDG-PET/CT was used for response assessment in a group of patients with MDR-TB at 2 months following treatment initiation [30]. FDG uptake in TB lesions was quantified using total glycolytic activity (TGA), a sum of the SUV of all TB lesions in individual patients. A change between TGA of lesions obtained at baseline and 2 months since initiation of treatment was used to predict treatment outcome. Majority of patients with successful treatment (and probably successful) outcome had a significant drop ($\geq$50%) in TGA at 2 months after therapy initiation. All the patients who adhered to treatment but eventually had treatment failure had either a rise or minimal change in TGA. FDG-PET/CT at 2 months was better at predicting treatment outcome compared with liquid culture at 2 months. This study done in a trial setting clearly shows the superiority of FDG-PET/CT imaging over the standard of care to predict treatment outcome [30].

Martin and colleagues recently evaluated the utility of FDG-PET/CT obtained at 2 months and the end of treatment in a cohort of HIV-infected patients with PTB and EPTB [31]. On 2-month FDG-PET/CT scans, 14/18 patients showed $\geq$a 20% decrease in the SUVmax of lesions representing a response to treatment.

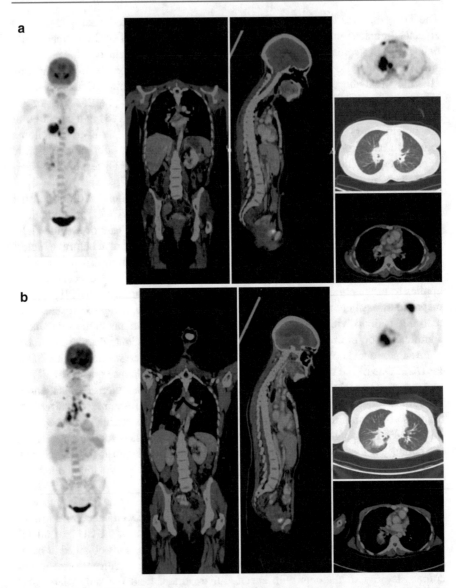

Fig. 11.1 FDGPET/CT shows mixed response to antituberculous therapy: A 41-year-old female with TB involvement of both lungs and mediastinal nodes. FDGPET/CT was obtained prior to treatment for baseline assessment (**a**). Follow-up FDG-PET/CT (**b**) Obtained 2 months after initiation of treatment showed response in the initial lesions with appearance of new sites nodal mediastinal nodal involvement

End-of-treatment (EOT) PET showed a further decline in SUVmax of TB lesions with 7/18 patients showing complete PET response while residual metabolically active lesions were seen in 8/18 patients. In these eight patients with residual metabolically active lesions, 14 of these lesions were nodal. In the group studied in this report, reactive lymphadenopathy due to HIV infection commonly demonstrated metabolic activity (mostly symmetrical), which may be a significant confounder in FDG-PET interpretation [32, 33]. It is, therefore, unknown the proportion of these lymph nodes that represent true residual disease due to TB lymphadenitis and a false-positive assessment due to HIV-associated reactive lymphadenopathy. The pattern of HIV-associated reactive lymphadenopathy as different from pathological nodal disease (due to infection such as TB or malignancy) has been evaluated in various studies. Early HIV infection is associated with lymphadenopathy in the neck, axillae, and mediastinum. As HIV infection progresses, HIV-associated lymphadenopathy commonly becomes generalized with the involvement of the groins. Chronic HIV infection is frequently associated with deep lymphadenopathy such as para-aortic retroperitoneal lymph node station [34]. The level of FDG uptake in HIV-associated reactive lymphadenopathy is directly related to the HIV viral load and inversely associated with the CD4+ T-cell count [35, 36].

Sathekge and colleagues, in 2011, demonstrated the ability of baseline FDG-PET/CT to predict treatment response in HIV-infected patients treated with standard ATT [37]. Non-responders tended to have involvement in multiple lymph node groups compared with responders. Involvement of ≥ 5 lymph node groups was a good predictor of treatment failure with a sensitivity, specificity, positive predictive value, and negative predictive value of 88%, 81%, 70%, and 93%, respectively. In another study by the same group done among HIV-infected patients with tuberculous lymphadenitis, SUVmax of involved lymph nodes on FDG-PET/CT obtained at 4 months after initiation of treatment was significantly higher in non-responders compared with responders (11.2 ± 4.0 versus 2.6 ± 2.8, $p = 0.0001$) [38]. A SUVmax of 4.5 in involved lymph nodes was able to separate responders from non-responders with a sensitivity, specificity, and accuracy of 88%, 85%, and 96% respectively. These early studies clearly show that despite the challenges inherent in FDG-PET assessment of lymph node involvement among the HIV-infected population, this imaging modality is still highly useful and outperform standalone morphologic imaging in this high-risk patient population [37, 38].

In a follow-up study to the ones by Sathekge et al., Lefebvre et al., in 2017, reported their findings among 18 patients with tuberculous lymphadenitis (mostly HIV-uninfected) evaluated with FDG-PET/CT obtained before or after completion of treatment for response assessment [39]. Half of the study patients had no residual metabolic activity and remained cured over a median follow-up period of about 2 years. Of these, five out of seven patients who had residual metabolic activity on EOT FDG-PET were cured including three patients who went on to have a negative follow-up FDG-PET/CT without additional treatment. Treatment was prolonged in two patients with PET findings considered to be partial response to treatment. While the study by Lefebvre and colleagues shows the excellent negative predictive value of FDG-PET/CT (none of the patients with negative PET experienced relapse) obtained before or at completion of treatment in assessing durable cure of TB lymphadenitis, it again brings to the fore, now in HIV-uninfected individuals, the clinical significance of residual metabolic activity in treated TB lesions. It remains to be determined the extent of residual metabolic activity that should be considered clinically significant requiring further treatment. Figure 11.2 shows FDG-PET/CT images of a patients with a negative EOT scan who remained without disease relapse more than 2 years after.

Stelzmueller et al. obtained 88 FDG-PET/CT scans at variable time points in 35 patients with PTB and EPTB for baseline and treatment response assessment [40]. Baseline FDG-PET showed more sites of disease involvement than CT. In 15 patients PET images showed complete metabolic response, while 16 and 4 patients had residual metabolic activity and new sites of disease involvement, respectively. The bone is a common site of EPTB involvement. TB involvement of the bone requires a prolonged treatment duration. Repeated biopsy for response assessment is impractical. Morphologic imaging with MRI, while very useful for the initial evaluation, maybe less so in the context of response assessment as morphologic improvement may trailed behind a microbiological cure. Dureja et al. demonstrated the clinical utility of FDG-PET/CT as a noninvasive imaging biomarker for response assessment in 33 patients with skeletal tuberculosis. FDG-PET/CT was obtained at baseline, 6, 12, and 18 months [41]. F-18 FDG-PET images show a progressive decline in SUV representing a response to ATT. The decline in SUV correlated well with clinical symptom (pain assessed on the visual analog scale) at 6 and 12 months since initiation of therapy but not with ESR [41]. Figure 11.3 shows the images of a patient whose treatment for TB spine was prolonged based on FDG-PET/CT findings.

11.3   The Significance of Residual Metabolic Activity Following Antituberculous Therapy

Patients considered cured based on clinical evaluation and negative mycobacterial culture often have residual lesions seen on imaging (Fig. 11.4). For morphological imaging, specific findings have been recognized to represent old, healed TB and do not connote active infection. Lesions considered to represent old, healed TB lesions include calcification of the involved organ such as lung, pleural, pericardial, and

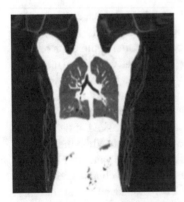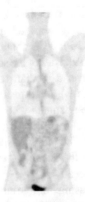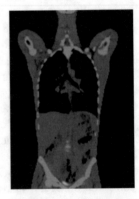

Fig. 11.2 FDG-PET/CT demonstrates excellent negative predictive value: A 35-year-old male who completed 6 months of standard anti-TB treatment. FDGPET/CT was obtained at the completion of treatment. Multiple bilateral pulmonary cysts without FDG uptake are seen. The patient remained cured after 2 years of follow-up

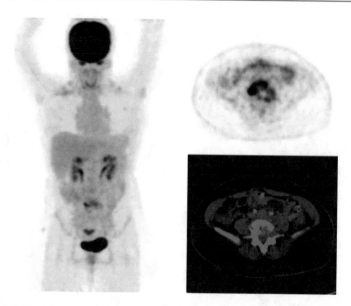

Fig. 11.3 FDGPET/CT is useful for the evaluation of adequacy of therapy: A 32-year-old female with TB in spine. After 12 months of anti-TB treatment, patient still had back pain. FDGPET/CT was obtained to evaluate for residual disease. Images show metabolic activity with destruction of L4 and L5 vertebrae associated with a para-spinal mass lesion all in favor of active residual TB lesion

nodal calcifications; fibrosis; lung cavitary changes; emphysematous changes; etc. [19]. Jeong and colleagues have reported FDG uptake in old, healed TB lesions [42]. ATT is most efficient in eliminating actively dividing bacilli. A subset of bacilli, however, only divide slowly or remain dormant. ATT is less effective in eradicating these slowly dividing and dormant bacilli and are implicated in causing disease relapse [28]. Persisting bacilli are nonculturable (negative mycobacterial culture) but remain minimally metabolically active [43]. Their presence stimulates antigenic and inflammatory reactions which may explain FDG uptake in old, healed TB lesions containing these bacilli. This was demonstrated recently in a large multinational study where FDG uptake was demonstrated in TB lesions of patients considered bacteriological cured [44]. Presence of replicating *Mycobacterium tuberculosis* (MTB) in these culture-negative patients was confirmed by the demonstration of MTB mRNA in the bronchoalveolar lavage samples obtained from the patients.

11.4 FDG-PET Quantitative Parameters for Response Assessment

Therapy response assessment is done either qualitatively or quantitatively. Qualitative assessment involves visual evaluation of TB lesions for FDG uptake in relation to background activity in normal organs/blood pool. Qualitative method of assessment lacks standardization and suffers from high interobserver variability.

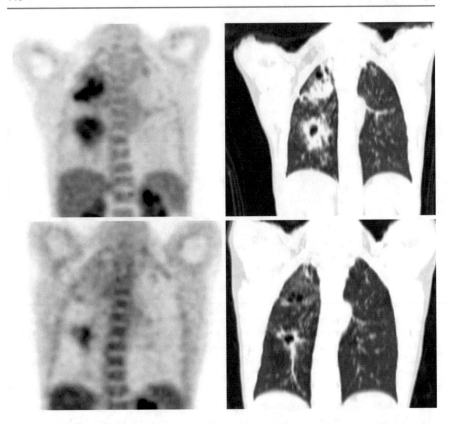

Fig. 11.4 Residual metabolically active TB lesion on end-of-treatment FDG-PET/CT is predictive of relapse: A 55-year-old female had baseline (top row) and end-of-treatment (bottom row) FDG PET/CT for the evaluation of pulmonary tuberculosis. Baseline scan shows two metabolically active fibro-cavitary lesions in the right lung. End-of-treatment scan showed residual metabolic activity in one of the baseline lesions. The patient experienced relapse 5 months after completion of TB treatment

SUV parameters, semiquantitative methods of quantifying FDG uptake in a lesion, are the most used quantification parameters for response assessment. SUVmax is the most commonly used SUV parameter with a lesser interobserver variability compared with visual assessment. No verified SUVmax cutoff that differentiates clinically significant FDG uptake in residual TB lesion at the end of treatment from those that are not clinically significant. Clinically insignificant FDG uptake in TB lesion will include low-grade uptake due to the presence of antigenic stimulation caused by dead or dying bacilli.

Metabolic lesion volume (MLV) and total lesion glycolysis (TLG) are SUV-based quantitative parameters most commonly used in oncologic imaging for quantification and prognostication [45–47]. They reflect the rate of glycolysis in a lesion as well as the volume of the lesion that is metabolically active (as against regions of necrosis and fibrosis). They reflect lesion biology better than SUVmax. MLV and TLG are now being used for lesion characterization and therapy outcome assessment in PET imaging of infectious diseases [48]. These parameters may prove to be more useful for predicting treatment outcome of TB in the future.

Artificial intelligence is making an inroad into image interpretation, quantification, and prognostication. Malherbe et al., in a recent pilot study, reported their findings with the use of an MLV and TLG-based semiautomatic algorithm for segmentation and quantification of complex TB lesions [49]. The technique which uses PET and CT criteria was able to track changes in TB lesion in response to treatment over time. Many of this type of computer-based image interpretation and prediction algorithm are becoming commonplace and may become clinically translatable in the near future.

11.5   Limitations of FDG-PET/CT for Response Assessment

The PET system has an inherent limitation in its spatial resolution which underestimates FDG avidity of lesions below twice its spatial resolution due to partial volume averaging. Improvement in PET technology is addressing this limitation with the newer PET systems having better spatial resolution. Certain organs like the brain and the heart have definite or variable intense physiologic FDG accumulation limiting the utility of FDG-PET for response assessment of TB involvement of these organs. Immune reconstitution syndrome is seen in individuals with MTB and HIV coinfection upon initiation of antiretroviral therapy [50]. This syndrome is characterized by worsening of clinical symptoms and an increase in FDG uptake in inflammatory lesions including TB. FDG-PET for response assessment must be planned with this treatment-related syndrome in mind. It remains to be determined which level of FDG uptake remaining in TB patients at the completion of treatment should be considered clinically significant. FDG was initially used for oncologic imaging and is not specific for TB. FDG avidity in lesions seen in patients evaluated for TB is not confirmatory of disease involvement. Studies reporting on the clinical utility of FDG-PET/CT for response assessment in TB are highly variable in their design, mostly have small study populations, and are therefore difficult to combine in a meta-analysis [51].

11.6   Conclusion

FDG-PET/CT performed during and at the completion of treatment is an accurate imaging marker for treatment response assessment in PTB and EPTB. It has excellent negative predictive value as patients who have complete resolution of disease at the end of treatment rarely experience a relapse. This often correlates with the clinical response and outperforms standalone morphologic imaging for response assessment.

References

1. Wu S, Zhang Y, Sun F, Chen M, Zhou L, Wang N, et al. Adverse events associated with the treatment of multi-drug-resistant tuberculosis: a systematic review and meta-analysis. Am J Ther. 2016;23(2):e521–30.
2. Senousy BE, Belal SI, Draganov PV. Hepatotoxic effects of therapies for tuberculosis. Nat Rev Gastroenterol Hepatol. 2010;7(10):543–56.
3. Krasniqi S, Jakupi A, Daci A, Tigani B, Jupoli-Krasniqi N, Pira M, et al. Tuberculosis treatment adherence of patients in Kosovo. Tuberc Res Treat. 2017;2017:4850324.
4. Ukwaja KN, Alobu I, Lgwenyi C, Hopewell PC. The high cost of free tuberculosis services: patient and household costs associated with tuberculosis care in Ebonyi State, Nigeria. PLoS One. 2013;8(8):e73134.
5. Pooran A, Pieterson E, Davids M, Theron G, Dheda K. What is the cost of diagnosis and management of drug resistant tuberculosis in South Africa? PLoS One. 2013;8(1):e54587.
6. Svensson EM, Svensson RJ, Te Brake LHM, Boeree MJ, Heinrich N, Konsten S, et al. The potential for treatment shortening with higher rifampicin doses: relating drug exposure to treatment response in patients with pulmonary tuberculosis. Clin Infect Dis. 2018;67(1):34–41.
7. Lambert ML, Hasker E, Van Deun A, Roberfroid D, Boelaert M, Van der Stuyft P. Recurrence in tuberculosis: relapse or re-infection? Lancet Infect Dis. 2003;3(5):282–7.
8. Gillespie SH, Crook AM, McHugh TD, Mendel CM, Meredith SK, Murray SR, et al. Four-month moxifloxacin-based regimens for drug-sensitive tuberculosis. N Engl J Med. 2014;371(17):1577–87.
9. Yeager H Jr, Lacy J, Smith LR, LeMaistre CA. Quantitative studies of mycobacterial populations in sputum and saliva. Am Rev Respir Dis. 1967;95(6):998–1004.
10. Kang HK, Jeong BH, Lee H, Park HY, Jeon K, Huh HJ, et al. Clinical significance of smear positivity for acid-fast bacilli after ≥5 months of treatment in patients with drug-susceptible pulmonary tuberculosis. Medicine (Baltimore). 2016;95:31.
11. Wright PW, Wallace RJ Jr, Wright NM, Brown BA, Griffith DE. Sensitivity of fluorochrome microscopy for detection of *Mycobacterium tuberculosis* versus nontuberculous mycobacteria. J Clin Microbiol. 1998;36(4):1046–9.
12. Van der Kuyp F, Mahan CS. Prolonged positivity of sputum smears with negative cultures during treatment for pulmonary tuberculosis. Int J Tuberc Lung Dis. 2012;2012(16):1663–7.
13. Phillips PPJ, Mendel CM, Nunn AJ, McHugh TD, Crook AM, Hunt R, et al. A comparison of liquid and solid culture for determining relapse and durable cure in phase III TB trials for new regimens. BMC Med. 2017;15(1):207.
14. Cudahy PGT, Warren JL, Cohen T, Wilson D. Trends in C-reactive protein, D-dimer, and fibrinogen during therapy for HIV-associated multidrug-resistant tuberculosis. Am J Trop Med Hyg. 2018;99(5):1336–41.
15. Wallis RS, Doherty TM, Onyebujoh P, Vahedi M, Laang H, Olesen O, et al. Biomarkers for tuberculosis disease activity, cure, and relapse. Lancet Infect Dis. 2009;9:162–72.
16. Mori T. Usefulness of interferon-gamma release assays for diagnosing TB infection and problems with these assays. J Infect Chemother. 2009;15(3):143–55.
17. Friedrich SO, Rachow A, Saathoff E, Singh K, Mangu CD, Dawson R, et al. Assessment of the sensitivity and specificity of Xpert MTB/RIF assays as an early sputum biomarker for response to tuberculosis treatment. Lancet Respir Med. 2013;1:462–70.
18. Skoura E, Zumla A, Bomanji J. Imaging in tuberculosis. Int J Infect Dis. 2015;32:87–93.
19. Hicks A, Muthukumarasamy S, Maxwell D, Howlett D. Chronic inactive pulmonary tuberculosis and treatment sequelae: chest radiographic features. Int J Tuberc Lung Dis. 2014;18(2):128–33.
20. Seon HJ, Kim YI, Lim SC, Kim YH, Kwon YS. Clinical significance of residual lesions in chest computed tomography after anti-tuberculosis treatment. Int J Tuberc Lung Dis. 2014;18(3):341–6.

21. Vorster M, Sathekge MM, Bomanji J. Advances in imaging of tuberculosis: the role of ^{18}F-FDG PET and PET/CT. Curr Opin Pulm Med. 2014;20(3):287–93.
22. Lawal I, Zeevaart JR, Ebenhan T, Ankrah A, Vorster M, Kruger HG, et al. Metabolic imaging of infection. J Nucl Med. 2017;58(11):1727–32.
23. Lawal I, Sathekge M. F-18 FDG PET/CT imaging of cardiac and vascular inflammation and infection. Br Med Bull. 2016;120(1):55–74.
24. Liu PT, Modlin RL. Human macrophage host defense against Mycobacterium tuberculosis. Curr Opin Immunol. 2008;20(4):371–6.
25. Ankrah AO, van der Werf TS, de Vries EF, Dierckx RA, Sathekge MM, Glaudemans AW. PET/CT imaging of Mycobacterium tuberculosis infection. Clin Transl Imaging. 2016;4:131–44.
26. Ankrah AO, Glaudemans AWJM, Maes A, Van de Wiele C, Dierckx RAJO, Vorster M, et al. Tuberculosis. Semin Nucl Med. 2018;48(2):108–30.
27. Lin PL, Coleman T, Carney JP, Lopresti BJ, Tomko J, Filmore D, et al. Radiologic responses in Cynomolgus macaques for assessing tuberculosis chemotherapy regimens. Antimimicrob Agents Chemother. 2013;57(9):4237–44.
28. Sathekge MM, Ankrah AO, Lawal I, Vorster M. Monitoring response to therapy. Semin Nucl Med. 2017;48(2):166–81.
29. Martinez V, Castilla-Lievre MA, Guillet-Caruba C, Grenier G, Fior R, Desarnaud S, et al. ^{18}F-FDG PET/CT in tuberculosis: an early non-invasive marker of therapeutic response. Int J Tuberc Lung Dis. 2012;16(9):1180–5.
30. Chen RY, Dodd LE, Lee M, Paripati P, Hammoud DA, Mountz JM, et al. PET/CT and high resolution CT as potential imaging biomarkers associated with treatment outcomes in MDR-TB. Sci Transl Med. 2014;6(265):265ra166.
31. Martin C, Castaigne C, Vierasu I, Garcia C, Wyndham-Thomas C, de Wit S. Prospective Serail FDG PET/CT during treatment of Extrapulmonary tuberculosis in HIV-infected patients: an exploratory study. Clin Nucl Med. 2018;43(9):635–40.
32. Mhlanga JC, Durand D, Tsai HL, Durand CM, Leal JP, Wang H, et al. Differentiation of HIV-associated lymphoma from HIV-associated reactive lymphadenopathy using quantitative PET and symmetry. Eur J Nucl Med Mol Imaging. 2014;41(4):596–604.
33. Sathekge M, Maes A, Van de Wiele C. FDG-PET in HIV infection and tuberculosis. Semin Nucl Med. 2013;43(5):349–66.
34. Iyengar S, Chin B, Margolick JB, Sabundayo BP, Schwartz DH. Anatomical loci of HIV-associated immune activation and association with viremia. Lancet. 2003;362(9388):945–50.
35. Lucignani G, Orunesu E, Cesari M, Marzo K, Pacei M. Bechi get al. FDG-PET imaging in HIV-infected subjects: relation with therapy and immunovirological variables. Eur J Nucl Med Mol Imaging. 2009;36(4):640–7.
36. Sathekge M, Maes A, Kgomo M, Van de Wiele C. Fluorodeoxyglucose uptake by lymph nodes of HIV patients is inversely related to CD4 cell count. Nucl Med Commun. 2010;31(2):137–40.
37. Sathekge M, Maes A, Kgomo M, Stoltz A, Van de Wiele C. Use of ^{18}F-FDG PET to predict response to first-line tuberculostatics in HIV-associated tuberculosis. J Nucl Med. 2011;52(6):880–5.
38. Sathekge M, Maes A, D'Asseler Y, Vorster M, Gongxeka H, Van de Wiele C. Tuberculous lymphadenitis: FDG PET and CT findings in responsive and nonresponsive disease. Eur J Nucl Med Mol Imaging. 2012;39(7):1184–90.
39. Lefebvre N, Argemi X, Meyer N, Mootien J, Douiri N, Sferrazza-Mandala S, et al. Clinical usefulness of ^{18}F-FDG PET/CT for initial staging and assessment of treatment efficacy in patients with lymph node tuberculosis. Nucl Med Biol. 2017;50:17–24.
40. Stelzmueller I, Huber H, Wunn R, Hodolic M, Mandl M, Lamprecht B, et al. ^{18}F-FDG PET/CT in the initial assessment and for follow-up in patients with tuberculosis. Clin Nucl Med. 2016;41(4):e187–94.
41. Dureja S, Sen IB, Acharya S. Potential role of F18 FDG PET-CT as an imaging biomarker for the noninvasive evaluation in uncomplicated skeletal tuberculosis: a prospective clinical observational study. Eur Spine J. 2014;23(11):2449–54.

42. Jeong YJ, Paeng JC, Nam HY, Lee JS, Lee SM, Yoo CG, et al. ^{18}F-FDG positron-emission tomography/computed tomography findings of radiographic lesions suggesting old healed tuberculosis. J Korean Med Sci. 2014;29(3):386–91.

43. Hu Y, Mangan JA, Dhillon J, Sole KM, Mitchison DA, Butcher PD, et al. Detection of mRNA transcripts and active transcription in persistent Mycobacterium tuberculosis induced by exposure to rifampin or pyrazinamide. J Bacteriol. 2000;182(22):6358–65.

44. Malherbe ST, Shenai S, Ronacher K, Loxton AG, Dolganov G, Kriel M, et al. Persisting positron emission tomography lesion activity and *Mycobacterium tuberculosis* mRNA after tuberculosis cure. Nat Med. 2016;22(10):1094–100.

45. Lawal IO, Ankrah AO, Mokoala KMG, Popoola GO, Kaoma CA, Maes A, et al. Prognostic value of pre-treatment F-18 FDG PET metabolic metrics in patients with locally advanced carcinoma of the anus with and without HIV infection. Nuklearmedizin. 2018;57(5):190–7.

46. Van de Wiele C, Kruse V, Smeets P, Sathekge M, Maes A. Predictive and prognostic value of metabolic tumour volume and total lesion glycolysis in solid tumours. Eur J Nucl Med Mol Imaging. 2013;40(2):290–301.

47. Lawal IO, Nyakale NE, Harry LM, Modiselle MR, Ankrah AO, Msomi AP, et al. The role of F-18 FDG PET/CT in evaluating the impact of HIV infection on tumor burden and therapy outcome in patients with Hodgkin lymphoma. Eur J Nucl Med Mol Imaging. 2017;44(12):2025–33.

48. Ankrah AO, Span LFR, Klein HC, de Jong PA, Dierckx RAJO, Kwee TC, et al. Role of FDG PET/CT in monitoring treatment response in patients with invasive fungal infection. Eur J Nucl Med Mol Imaging. 2019;46(1):174–83.

49. Malherbe ST, Dupont P, Kant I, Ahlers P, Kriel M, Loxton AG, et al. Semi-automatic technique to quantify complex tuberculous lung lesions on ^{18}F-fluorodeoxyglucose positron emission tomography/computerized tomography images. EJNMMI Res. 2018;8:55.

50. Hammoud DA, Boulougoura A, Papadakis GZ, Wang J, Dodd LE, Rupert A, et al. Increased metabolic activity on F-Fluorodeoxyglucose positron emission tomography-computed tomography in human immunodeficiency virus-associated immune reconstitution inflammatory syndrome. Clin Infect Dis. 2019;68(2):229–38.

51. Sjölander H, Strørn T, Gerke O, Hess S. Value of FDG-PET/CT for treatment response in tuberculosis: a systematic review and meta-analysis. Clin Transl Imaging. 2018;6(1):19–29.

Non-FDG PET Tracers for TB Imaging

12

T. Ebenhan and Mariza Vorster

Contents

12.1 Introduction

PET/CT imaging provides a noninvasive whole-body molecular imaging tool, and TB imaging with FDG has been gradually establishing itself in the settings of detection of especially extrapulmonary disease involvement as well as in the monitoring of treatment response. However, ^{18}F-FDG-PET/CT imaging still suffers from several limitations, which creates the need for non-FDG PET tracers. These include such factors as the need for a nearby cyclotron, the cost of ^{18}F-FDG, the non-specificity thereof, and the normal biodistribution that limits disease detection in especially the brain, the gastrointestinal, and genitourinary tracts.

The pathophysiology of *M. tuberculosis* also presents a number of distinctive challenges to tracer design. Replication of *M. tuberculosis* can range from totally dormant to as rapid division as every 18 h in vivo, which renders tracers inefficient if such tracers accumulate due to cell cycle activity. Mycobacteria also have the

T. Ebenhan (✉) · M. Vorster
Department of Nuclear Medicine, University of Pretoria & Steve Biko Academic Hospital, Pretoria, South Africa

© Springer Nature Switzerland AG 2020
D. Sobic Saranovic et al. (eds.), *PET/CT in Tuberculosis*, Clinicians' Guides to Radionuclide Hybrid Imaging, https://doi.org/10.1007/978-3-030-47009-8_12

ability to form part of compounded pathological structures, such as tuberculomas, which may hinder results when using nonspecific nuclear imaging techniques [1]. For a TB-imaging tracer it would be paramount to achieve sufficient penetration into the tuberculoma which may be additionally complicated if imaging of engulfed bacteria is the targeting approach.

Although imaging with PET/CT is unlikely to establish a routine role in the clinical work-up of patients with TB in the near future, it may provide useful information concerning the following:

- Distinguishing active from inactive disease
- Identification of individuals with latent disease who are at a high risk of developing reactivation of TB
- Identification of sites and disease extent in Extra-pulmonary Tuberculosis
- Determination of treatment response

The underlying pathophysiology and intended therapeutic drugs provide various targets for such imaging. Although there is a multitude of tracer possibilities, this chapter will start with an outline of some of the most recent developments in terms of preclinical and research targets, and then focus on a few of the tracers that have been successfully applied in a reasonable number of patients.

12.2   Research/ Preclinical Tracers

The last decade of research in molecular imaging has revealed great potential for novel imaging agents and candidates for TB [2]. Those tracers (Table 12.1) may be categorized as follows: (a) radio-biomimetics, (b) radiolabeled antibodies or peptides, and (c) radiolabeled antitubercular drugs.

The use of biomimetics as new radiopharmaceuticals followed the approach of ^{18}F-FDG but these tracers are more specific for *M. tuberculosis* or bacteria-harboring host cells. For instance, N,N-diethyl-2-(4-methoxyphenyl)-5,7-dimethylpyrazolo[1,5-a]pyrimidine-3-acetamide (DPA-713), a carbon-11- or iodine-125-radiolabeled ligand of the translocator protein (TSPO), demonstrated selective accumulation within macrophages and phagocytic cells. This allowed for single-photon emission computed tomography (SPECT)/PET imaging of TB-associated inflammatory lesions (Fig. 12.1) with a superior retention index over ^{18}F-FDG [3, 4]. A better understanding of the tuberculoma substructures revealed regions of necrosis and hypoxia [5]. These findings were confirmed in vivo using ^{64}copper(II)-diacetyl-bis(N^4-methylthiosemicarbazone) (^{64}Cu-ATSM)- and ^{18}F-fluoromisonidazole (^{18}F-FMISO)-PET demonstrating that tissues surrounding pulmonary cavities in patients with TB were indeed hypoxic [6]. Furthermore, sodium(^{18}F)fluoride-PET was capable of imaging microcalcifications of TB lesions in a chronically *M. tuberculosis*–infected murine model [7]. Other biomimetics including the bacteria unique disaccharide trehalose [8] and its deoxyfluoro-D-derivative [9] were ^{18}F-fluorinated recently to allow for PET imaging of *M. tuberculosis*–infected animals.

The molecule PT70 (5-Hexyl-2-(2-methylphenoxy)phenol) is a diaryl ether inhibitor of InhA, the enoyl-ACP reductase in the *Mycobacterium tuberculosis* fatty

Table 12.1 Preclinical/research tracers

Tracer	Radio-isotope	Target	Class	References
DPA-713	[^{18}F]	Translocator protein	Radio-biomimetic	[3, 4]
ATSM	[^{64}Cu]	TB lesion hypoxia	Radio-biomimetic	[6]
FMISO	[^{18}F]	TB lesion hypoxia	Radio-biomimetic	[5]
Sodium fluoride	[^{18}F]	TB lesion microcalcification	Radio-biomimetic	[7]
Trehalose	[^{18}F]	Mycolic acid synthesis	Radio-biomimetic	[8]
Deoxyfluoro-D-trehalose	[$^{18/19}$F]	Mycolic acid synthesis	Radio-biomimetic	[9]
PT70	[^{11}C]	Enoyl-ACP reductase	Radio-biomimetic	[10]
FIAU	[^{18}F]	Bacterial thymidine kinase	Radio-biomimetic	[11]
TBIA101	[^{68}Ga]	TB-associated inflammation	Radio-peptide	[12]
Isoniazid	[^{11}C], [^{18}F]	Enoyl-ACP reductase	Radio-drug	[13, 14]
Rifampin	[^{11}C]	DNA-dependent RNA PM	Radio-drug	[13, 15]
Pyrazinamide	[^{11}C], [^{18}F]	Pyrazinamidase	Radio-drug	[13, 16]

DPA-713 N,N-diethyl-2-(4-methoxyphenyl)-5,7-dimethylpyrazolo[1,5-a]pyrimidine-3-acetamide, *ATSM* Copper(II)-diacetyl-bis(N^4-methylthiosemicarbazone), *FMISO* fluoromisonidazole, *PT70* 5-Hexyl-2-(2-methylphenoxy)phenol, *FIAU* 1-(−2-deoxy-2-fluoro-1-beta-D-arabino-furanosyl)-5-iodouracil, *TBIA101* PLPVLTI-GG-1,4,7,10-tetraazacyclododecane-1,4,7,10-tetraacetic acid, *TB* tuberculosis, *DNA* deoxyribonucleic acid, *RNA* ribonucleic acid, *PM* polymerase, *ACP* acyl carrier protein

acid biosynthesis pathway. It has a residence time of 24 min on the target, and also shows antibacterial activity in a mouse model of tuberculosis infection. Due to the interest in studying target tissue pharmacokinetics of PT70, researchers developed a method to ^{11}C-radiolabel PT70 and have studied its pharmacokinetics in mice and baboons using PET [10]. The nucleotide analogue FIAU (1-(2′-deoxy-2′-fluoro-beta-D-arabinofuranosyl)-5-iodouracil) is a selective substrate of bacterial thymidine kinase which can phosphorylate $^{123/4/5}$I- or ^{18}F-FIAU; thereby trapping this tracer and allowing it to accumulate in the bacteria. Wild-type *M. tuberculosis* does not express TK; however, genetically altered *M. tuberculosis* expressing TK has accumulated FIAU in experimentally infected animals [11].

Whereas most biomimetics are processed by *M. tuberculosis*' metabolizing machinery, radiolabeled antibodies and peptides are targeting the bacterial cell envelope. These molecules are well-studied biomarkers for several diseases, and great progress has been made to study bacterial infection. Due to the unique cell wall structure of *M. tuberculosis* no direct targeting agent from this class has been developed; however TBIA-101 is an example for host cell targeting agents that may detect inflammation using PET imaging. It is a 1,4,7,10-tetraazacyclododecane-1,4,7,10-tetraacetic

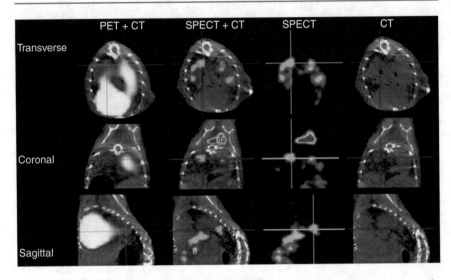

Fig. 12.1 [^{125}I]Iodo-DPA-713 localizes to tuberculosis lesions. The transverse, coronal, and sagittal images from a representative *Mycobacterium tuberculosis*–infected C3HeB/FeJ mouse that underwent both [^{125}I]iodo-DPA-713 single-photon emission computed tomography–high-resolution CT (SPECT-CT) and [^{18}F]FDG positron emission tomography (PET)–high-resolution CT are shown. Discrete areas of [^{125}I]iodo-DPA-713 SPECT signal are noted in the lungs of the infected mouse. The SPECT signal colocalizes with the tuberculosis lesion seen on CT (crosshair). The [^{18}F]FDG-PET signal is more diffuse, with intense signal noted in the heart, obscuring the pericardial regions. [^{125}I]iodo-DPA-713 SPECT signal is also noted in the brown fat (BF) in the coronal view

acid (^{68}Ga-DOTA)-functionalized depsipeptide (PLPVLTI) which showed promising uptake in *M. tuberculosis*–bearing rabbits. The findings suggest that ^{68}Ga-TBIA101-PET/CT may detect TB-associated inflammation, although more foundational studies need to be performed to rationalize the diagnostic value of this technique [12].

First-line TB drugs were developed to efficiently treat the disease; however, the structure of these drugs and their distinct targeting mechanism have raised interest to modify them to become radiopharmaceuticals. Li et al. ^{11}C-labeled isoniazid, rifampin, and pyrazinamide and studied their biodistribution in healthy baboons by way of PET imaging (See Fig. 12.2) [13]. The structural promiscuity of these molecules may allow for slight chemically modifications to replace ^{11}C (short radiochemical half-life) with longer half-life isotopes (e.g., ^{18}F) but not without thorough validation. In this fashion 2-^{18}F-fluoroisonicotinic acid hydrazide (2-^{18}F-INH), the fluoro-derivative of isoniazid, was developed and applied as a PET tracer for imaging *M. tuberculosis*-infected rodents. The validation of 2-^{18}F-INH as a marker of isoniazid distribution required verifying both that it accumulated intracellular like isoniazid and that it matched isoniazid in its mechanism of conversion from prodrug to active drug. Dynamic PET imaging demonstrated that 2-^{18}F-INH was extensively distributed, and rapidly accumulated at the sites of infection, including necrotic pulmonary TB granulomas (See Fig. 12.3) [14].

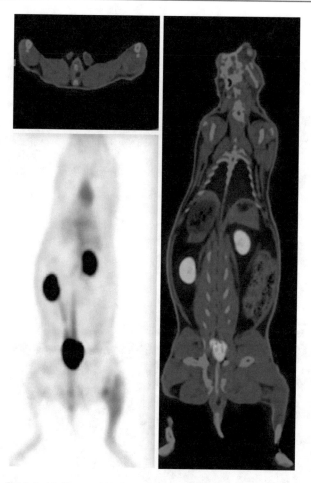

Fig. 12.2 Ga-68 labeled DOTA-TBIA101 visualizing inflammation due to muscular *M. tuberculosis* infection in rabbits (arrows indicate the infection slide on (**a**) PET MIP image, (**b**) an axial PET/CT slide, and (**c**) a coronal PET/CT slide)

DeMarco et al. recently performed dynamic microdose ^{11}C-rifampin-PET imaging to reveal differences in intralesional pharmacokinetics; thus, noninvasive imaging may be used to assess the distribution of drugs into compartments of interest, with potential applications for TB drug regimen development [15]. In 2017, 5-^{18}F-pyrazinamide (5-^{18}F-PZA) the ^{18}F-radiotracer analog of pyrazinamide, was employed to determine the biodistribution of 5-F-PZA using PET imaging and ex vivo analysis. Unfortunately, 5-^{18}F-PZA was not a substrate for pyrazinamidase, the bacterial enzyme that activates pyrazinamide, and the minimum inhibitory concentration (MIC) value for 5-F-PZA against *M. tuberculosis* was about 100-times higher than that for pyrazinamide [16].

The granuloma is central to the pathophysiology of tuberculosis and comprises of various immune cells that are representative of innate immunity and which at a later

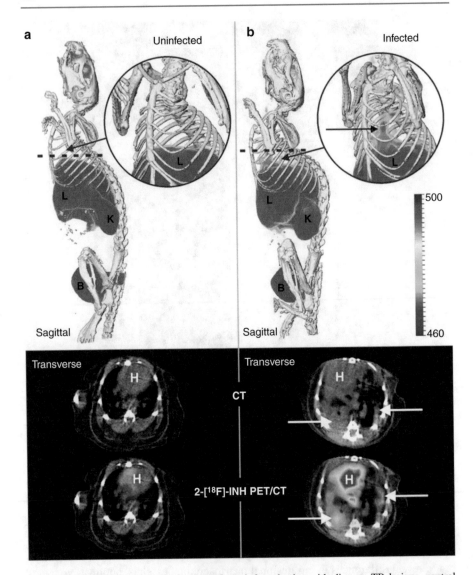

Fig. 12.3 PET/CT imaging of *M. tuberculosis*–infected mice with discrete TB lesions, central necrosis, and hypoxia. Uninfected (**a**) and infected (**b**) C3HeB/FeJ pairs were imaged after injection of 2-[¹⁸F]-FDG (**a**) or 2-[¹⁸F]-INH (**b**). Whole-animal sagittal and transverse sections are displayed as combined PET/CT images with heart (H), liver (L), kidneys (K), and bladder (B) marked. Discrete foci of 2-[¹⁸F]-INH-PET activity colocalizing with the TB lesions (as seen on CT) is noted in the lung fields of the infected (**b**) but not the uninfected mouse (**a**), suggesting that 2-[¹⁸F]-INH penetrates and concentrates at the site of TB lesions. Uptake in the heart, liver, kidneys, and bladder is noted in both infected and uninfected animals

stage stimulate the processes involved in adaptive immunity. TB granulomas are dynamic structures with lymphocyte movements that are similar to those found with lymph nodes. The early granulomas promote phagocytosis of infected macrophages and secrete MMP-9, which in turn stimulate chemotaxis of new macrophages. As such, it provides multiple targets for imaging [17]. Future TB granuloma imaging possibilities also include leukocyte-targeted peptide probes, such as reported on by Locke et al. [18] Cu-64-based imaging, such as ^{64}Cu-CB-TE K1P has also been used in the imaging of macrophages in TB granulomas as reported by Zeng et al. [19]

12.3 Tracers Used in Clinical Settings

12.3.1 ^{11}C/^{18}F-Choline

The mechanism of uptake of choline-based PET imaging (whether labeled to F-18 or C-11) is increased cell membrane metabolism, where it is biochemically indistinguishable from the natural form of choline as a component of cell membranes [20–22]. In tumor cells, the increased metabolism results in an increase in the uptake of choline to maintain the increasing demand for synthesis of phospholipids in cellular membranes. The use of ^{18}F-choline in the setting of prostate cancer is well known; however, several authors have also evaluated its use in other malignancies [20]. In the setting of chest pathology, Liu et al. (2006) investigated the role of ^{11}C-choline in the evaluation of middle mediastinal pathology and found an accuracy of 75% in distinguishing benign from malignant lesions [23], whereas Hara et al. (2000) found a 100% diagnostic accuracy of ^{11}C-choline in detecting mediastinal lymph node metastases from non-small cell lung cancer [24].

Choline imaging has also been applied in the setting of tuberculosis, and Hara et al. have published the majority of research in this setting. In their 2003 publication, 14 patients with pulmonary TB as well as 5 patients with atypical mycobacterial infections were included. The diagnosis of TB was confirmed with bacterial cultures and all patients underwent PET/CT imaging with both FDG and choline. The authors reported a relatively constant SUV of around 2, which was independent of lesion size and was significantly lower than that reported for FDG. This group suggested that the combination of imaging with FDG and choline could potentially help to distinguish lung cancer (which demonstrated high uptake on both studies) from tuberculosis (which demonstrated high uptake on FDG, but low uptake on choline) especially in the setting of solitary pulmonary nodules (SPN) [25].

The authors proposed that this pattern of uptake was associated with the presence of hard granulomas, representative of a more chronic phase of TB where the granuloma is composed mainly of clusters of macrophages with decreased or absent blood vessels. In these relatively hypoxic or anoxic tissue conditions, macrophages adapt to anaerobic glycolysis and the cell membranes are relatively non-proliferative. The aforementioned changes result in an increased uptake on FDG and relatively decreased uptake with choline [25].

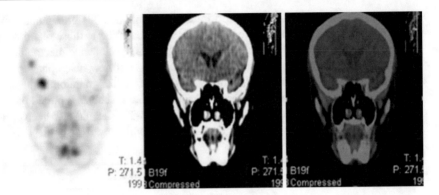

Fig. 12.4 ¹⁸F-Choline PET/CT imaging allows for detection of tuberculous brain involvement in the absence of normal biodistribution in this region

At our center in Pretoria, South Africa, we have demonstrated the advantage of imaging a TB patient with ¹⁸F-choline in a case with brain involvement (see Fig. 12.4). The brain involvement could be demonstrated more clearly on the choline image due to the absence of normal tracer biodistribution in this region [26].

12.3.2 ⁶⁸Ga-Citrate

The uptake mechanism of gallium is complex, incompletely understood, and involves several direct as well as indirect mechanisms. Local inflammation and vasodilation result in increased tracer accumulation due to higher tracer delivery (indirect), while direct mechanisms are the result of gallium's similarity to iron. Its accumulation in tuberculous lesions is believed to be the result of transcapillary exudation of transferrin-bound gallium and subsequent binding to leucocytes and bacteria. Gallium accumulation is therefore unaffected by the impaired cellular immunity found in patients with HIV [27].

Gallium scintigraphy (in the form of ⁶⁷Ga-citrate) has played an important role in the diagnosis and management of patients with TB and HIV as early as the 1970s. Sarkar et al. evaluated the use of ⁶⁷Ga-citrate imaging in 11 patients with suspected extrapulmonary involvement and found that it could correctly predict the absence or presence of active disease. They also suggested that ⁶⁷Ga-citrate should be routinely used in patients with suspected extrapulmonary involvement and that it would probably be valuable in the follow-up evaluation since scan findings correlated well with clinical improvement [28]. Several other authors have evaluated the use of gallium imaging in patients with immunosuppression and lung diseases, such as tuberculosis, reaching similar conclusions [29–31].

The rationale for imaging with ⁶⁸Ga-citrate includes the improved resolution, the year-round tracer availability from a generator, and followed on the success of its SPECT predecessor, gallium-67 citrate, in the setting of granulomatous diseases.

In a South African pilot study, 13 patients with tuberculosis were imaged with ⁶⁸Ga-citrate PET/CT. Findings demonstrated extrapulmonary involvement in 10 of these patients and suggested a possible distinction between areas of active and non-active disease. Extrapulmonary TB involvement included lymph nodes, bone, pleura, spleen, and gastrointestinal tract and ^{68}Ga-citrate PET/CT outperformed the detection capabilities of CT in this setting.

12.3.3 ^{18}F-FLT

Fluorothymidine (FLT) is a thymidine analogue, which follows the integration of thymidine into the bacterial DNA. FLT imaging has mainly been used as part of a combination of tracers in a multimodality imaging setting. Several groups have reported on its use in combination with ^{18}F-FDG-PET imaging to distinguish TB from malignant lesions in the lung and suggested a role in the diagnosis and management of pulmonary lesions [32, 33]. In a 2015 meta-analysis (consisting of 548 patients) on the performance of FLT-PET for pulmonary lesions as compared to FDG-PET, the authors concluded that imaging with FLT could potentially reduce the number of false-positive findings with FDG-PET in TB patients. FLT-PET imaging outperformed FDG in ruling out inflammatory lesions noted in patients with TB [34].

12.4   In Summary

- There are a vast number of preclinical/research tracers in development, which can be broadly categorized as follows: (a) radio-biomimetics, (b) radiolabeled antibodies or peptides, and (c) radiolabeled antitubercular drugs.
- Exciting potential TB-imaging options include granuloma-imaging possibilities such as leukocyte-targeted peptide probes, ^{64}Cu-based probes, hypoxia-imaging probes, and radiolabeled anti-TB drugs.
- Non-FDG-PET tracers with the greatest clinical potential (and often used in combination with ^{18}F-FDG) include ^{18}F/^{11}C-choline, ^{68}Ga-citrate, and ^{18}F-FLT.

References

1. D'Souza MM, Tripathi M, Shrivastav M, Sharma R, Mondal A. Tuberculosis mimicking malignancy. Hell J Nucl Med. 2009;12(1):69–70.
2. Johnson DH, Via LE, Kim P, et al. Nuclear imaging: a powerful novel approach for tuberculosis. Nucl Med Biol. 2014;41(10):777–84.
3. Ordonez AA, Pokkali S, DeMarco VP, et al. Radioiodinated DPA-713 imaging correlates with bactericidal activity of tuberculosis treatments in mice. Antimicrob Agents Chemother. 2015;59(1):642–9.
4. Foss CA, Harper JS, Wang H, Pomper MG, Jain SK. Noninvasive molecular imaging of tuberculosis-associated inflammation with radioiodinated DPA-713. J Infect Dis. 2013;208(12):2067–74.
5. Belton M, Brilha S, Manavaki R, et al. Hypoxia and tissue destruction in pulmonary TB. Thorax. 2016;71(12):1145–53.
6. Harper J, Skerry C, Davis SL, et al. Mouse model of necrotic tuberculosis granulomas develops hypoxic lesions. J Infect Dis. 2012;205(4):595–602.

7. Ordonez AA, DeMarco VP, Klunk MH, Pokkali S, Jain SK. Imaging chronic Tuberculous lesions using sodium [(18)F]Fluoride positron emission tomography in mice. Mol Imaging Biol. 2015;17(5):609–14.
8. Backus KM, Boshoff HI, Barry CS, et al. Uptake of unnatural trehalose analogs as a reporter for Mycobacterium tuberculosis. Nat Chem Biol. 2011;7(4):228–35.
9. Rundell SR, Wagar ZL, Meints LM, et al. Deoxyfluoro-d-trehalose (FDTre) analogues as potential PET probes for imaging mycobacterial infection. Org Biomol Chem. 2016;14(36):8598–609.
10. Wang H, Liu L, Lu Y, et al. Radiolabelling and positron emission tomography of PT70, a time-dependent inhibitor of InhA, the Mycobacterium tuberculosis enoyl-ACP reductase. Bioorg Med Chem Lett. 2015;25(21):4782–6.
11. Davis SL, Be NA, Lamichhane G, et al. Bacterial thymidine kinase as a non-invasive imaging reporter for Mycobacterium tuberculosis in live animals. PLoS One. 2009;4(7):e6297.
12. Ebenhan T, Mokaleng BB, Venter JD, Kruger HG, Zeevaart JR, Sathekge M. Preclinical assessment of a (68)Ga-DOTA-functionalized Depsipeptide as a Radiodiagnostic infection imaging agent. Molecules. 2017;22(9):1403.
13. Liu L, Xu Y, Shea C, Fowler JS, Hooker JM, Tonge PJ. Radiosynthesis and bioimaging of the tuberculosis chemotherapeutics isoniazid, rifampicin and pyrazinamide in baboons. J Med Chem. 2010;53(7):2882–91.
14. Weinstein EA, Liu L, Ordonez AA, et al. Noninvasive determination of 2-[18F]-fluoroisonicotinic acid hydrazide pharmacokinetics by positron emission tomography in Mycobacterium tuberculosis-infected mice. Antimicrob Agents Chemother. 2012;56(12):6284–90.
15. DeMarco VP, Ordonez AA, Klunk M, et al. Determination of [11C]rifampin pharmacokinetics within Mycobacterium tuberculosis-infected mice by using dynamic positron emission tomography bioimaging. Antimicrob Agents Chemother. 2015;59(9):5768–74.
16. Zhang Z, Ordonez AA, Smith-Jones P, et al. The biodistribution of 5-[18F]fluoropyrazinamide in Mycobacterium tuberculosis-infected mice determined by positron emission tomography. PLoS One. 2017;12(2):e0170871.
17. Ramakrishnan L. Revisiting the role of the granuloma in tuberculosis. Nat Rev Immunol. 2012;12(5):352.
18. Locke LW, Kothandaraman S, Tweedle M, Chaney S, Wozniak DJ, Schlesinger LS. Use of a leukocyte-targeted peptide probe as a potential tracer for imaging the tuberculosis granuloma. Tuberculosis. 2018;108:201–10.
19. Zeng D, Mattila J, Beaino W, Jiang M, Lopresti B, Coleman M, Flynn J, Anderson C. Copper-64-labeled CB-TE1K1P conjugates of MCP-1 for PET imaging of macrophages in tuberculosis granulomas. J Nucl Med. 2014;55(supplement 1):1210.
20. Treglia G, Giovannini E, Di Franco D, Calcagni ML, Rufini V, Picchio M, et al. The role of positron emission tomography using carbon-11 and fluorine-18 choline in tumors other than prostate cancer: a systematic review. Bull Cancer. 2012;26(6):451–61.
21. Peng ZZ, Liu QQ, Li MM, Han MM, Yao SS, Liu QQ. Comparison of (11)C-choline PET/CT and enhanced CT in the evaluation of patients with pulmonary abnormalities and locoregional lymph node involvement in lung cancer. Clin Lung Cancer. 2012;13(4):312–20.
22. Pieterman RM, Que TH, Elsinga PH, Pruim J, van Putten JWG, Willemsen ATM, et al. Comparison of 11C-choline and 18F-FDG PET in primary diagnosis and staging of patients with thoracic cancer. J Nucl Med. 2002;43(2):167–72.
23. Liu Q, Peng Z-M, Liu Q-W, Yao S-Z, Zhang L, Meng L, et al. The role of 11C-choline positron emission tomography-computed tomography and videomediastinoscopy in the evaluation of diseases of middle mediastinum. Chin Med J. 2006;119(8):634–9.
24. Hara T, Inagaki K, Kosaka N, Morita T. Sensitive detection of mediastinal lymph node metastasis of lung cancer with 11C-choline PET. J Nucl Med. 2000;41(9):1507–13.
25. Hara T, Kosaka N, Suzuki T, Kudo K, Niino H. Uptake rates of 18F-fluorodeoxyglucose and 11C-choline in lung cancer and pulmonary tuberculosis: a positron emission tomography study. Chest. 2003;124(3):893–901.

26. Vorster M, Stoltz A, Jacobs AG, Sathekge MM. Imaging of pulmonary tuberculosis with 18F-fluoro-deoxy-glucose and 18F-ethylcholine. Open Nucl Med J. 2014;6:17–21.
27. Tsan MF. Mechanism of gallium-67 accumulation in inflammatory lesions. J Nucl Med. 1985;26(1):88–92.
28. Sarkar SD, Ravikrishnan KP, Woodbury DH, Carson JJ, Daley K. Gallium-67 citrate scanning--a new adjunct in the detection and follow-up of extrapulmonary tuberculosis: concise communication. J Nucl Med. 1979;20(8):833–6.
29. Rubin RHR, Fischman AJA. Radionuclide imaging of infection in the immunocompromised host. Clin Infect Dis. 1996;22(3):414–23.
30. Bekerman C, Hoffer PB, Bitran JD, Gupta RG. Gallium-67 citrate imaging studies of the lung. Semin Nucl Med. 1980;10(3):286–301.
31. Santin M, Podzamczer D, Ricart I, Mascaro J, Ramon JM, Dominguez A, et al. Utility of the Gallium-67 citrate scan for the early diagnosis of tuberculosis in patients infected with the human immunodeficiency virus. Clin Infect Dis. 1995;20(3):652–6.
32. Xu B, Guan Z, Liu C, Wang R, Yin D, Zhang J, Chen Y, Yao S, Shao M, Wang H, Tian J. Can multimodality imaging using 18 F-FDG/18 F-FLT PET/CT benefit the diagnosis and management of patients with pulmonary lesions? Eur J Nucl Med Mol Imaging. 2011;38(2):285–92.
33. Tian J, Yang X, Yu L, Chen P, Xin J, Ma L, Feng H, Tan Y, Zhao Z, Wu W. A multicenter clinical trial on the diagnostic value of dual-tracer PET/CT in pulmonary lesions using 3'-deoxy-3'-18F-fluorothymidine and 18F-FDG. J Nucl Med. 2008;49:186–94.
34. Wang Z, Wang Y, Sui X, Zhang W, Shi R, Zhang Y, Dang Y, Qiao Z, Zhang B, Song W, Jiang J. Performance of FLT-PET for pulmonary lesion diagnosis compared with traditional FDG-PET: a meta-analysis. Eur J Radiol. 2015;84(7):1371–7.

Printed in the United States
By Bookmasters